MODERN BRITISH AMBULANCES

PETER MURPHY

D1464784

Bromley Libraries

30128 80307 944 4

First published 2017

Amberley Publishing
The Hill, Stroud
Gloucestershire, GL5 4EP

www.amberley-books.com

Copyright © Peter Murphy, 2017

The right of Peter Murphy to be identified as
the Author of this work has been asserted in
accordance with the Copyrights, Designs and
Patents Act 1988.

ISBN 978 1 4456 6788 1 (print)
ISBN 978 1 4456 6789 8 (ebook)

British Library Cataloguing in Publication Data.
A catalogue record for this book is available from
the British Library.

Origination by Amberley Publishing.
Printed in the UK.

Introduction

The modern British ambulance service has a variety of vehicles that form the backbone of emergency and medical transport. This book takes a look at the ambulances from the starting point, to the types of ambulances that were in service in the year 2000, and finally to the types of ambulance used to the present day. The front-line NHS ambulance is the vehicle that is most commonly associated with the ambulance service. As well as this, the NHS ambulance service have rapid response cars that get clinicians acting as solo responders to emergency calls to initiate treatment. For less urgent calls, patient transport ambulances are used for non-emergency patient transport, and hazardous-area response teams also have special vehicles for use in complex incidents. These all form part of the fleet that can be seen every day serving the public.

Taking a look just at the NHS is only half of the story of the modern British ambulance. With the growing number of private ambulance services now working in partnership with the NHS and undertaking specialist contract work, there are many different, and sometimes striking liveries seen on private ambulances. With the growing use of event medical cover having medical firms providing ambulances, these too have multiplied since 2000, and can often be seen in the summer months providing event cover. However, the more commonly associated voluntary aid societies also have a large presence in the British ambulance scene. While most ambulances are road-based, there are a number of air ambulances, there are a number of air ambulance charities that provide medical response and offer fast journeys to hospitals, which can often be vital for the patient. One final consideration is the lesser-used works ambulance, where large industrial sites have an ambulance that works around the grounds. All these have their part to play in responding to emergencies, taking people to and from hospital, and acting as a safety net.

The modern ambulance has a vital part to play in coming to the aid of those in need and on my travels these are some of the photos that I have taken, though my thanks go to Mr Chris Playforth and Mr Stuart McKenzie who have contributed photos to my collection and have been included in this book. These are a snapshot of the ambulances that have been employed in various places and in various uses. There are some designs that are now obsolete and others that can be seen still in service today.

One of the aims of my collection is to show that, alongside the traditional ambulance, the other varied types of vehicle are all part of the diverse and eclectic mixture that make up the modern British ambulance story.

My thanks go to all at Amberley Publishing, to my family and friends for their good wishes in producing this book, and also my profound thanks to my own ambulance colleagues – both former and current – and to all the other ambulance crews who have knowingly or unknowingly helped me in this photographic adventure.

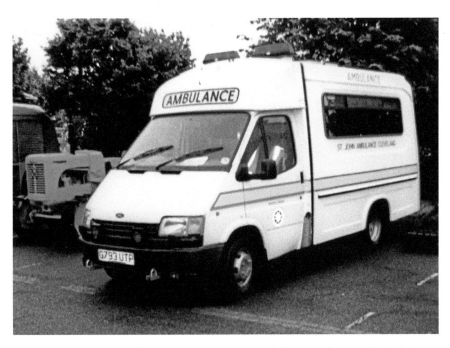

A 1989 Ford Transit/Wadham-Stringer MIAB (Modular Interchangeable Ambulance Body), (G793UTP), seen on 22 July 2001 when in use with St John Ambulance Cleveland on a public event duty. This ambulance was sold off soon after the photo was taken as St John Ambulance standardised their fleet nationally.

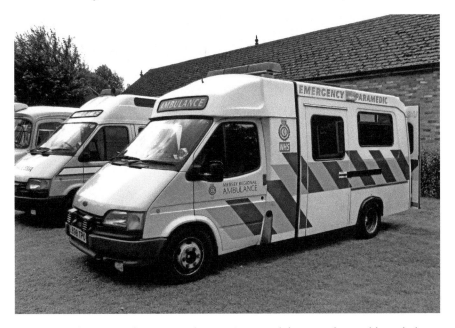

A 1993 Ford Transit MkIII/Customline MIAB. (Modular Interchangeable ambulance Body), (L698 TPO). A former Mersey Regional Ambulance Service frontline ambulance, it is now preserved. In service it was based at Northwich in Cheshire. A number of these ambulances were seeing their final days in service in the early 2000s.

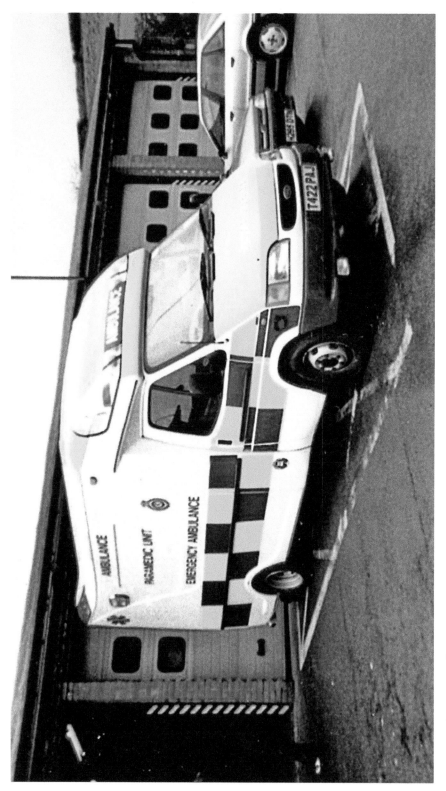

A 1999 Ford Transit/Wilker 'Luna', (T422PAJ), seen at Carlin How ambulance station on 22 May 2000 when in operational service with the Tees, East and North Yorkshire Ambulance Service NHS Trust. This was one of the first ambulances in their fleet to wear the 'Battenberg' livery at a time when ambulances were white with yellow fronts.

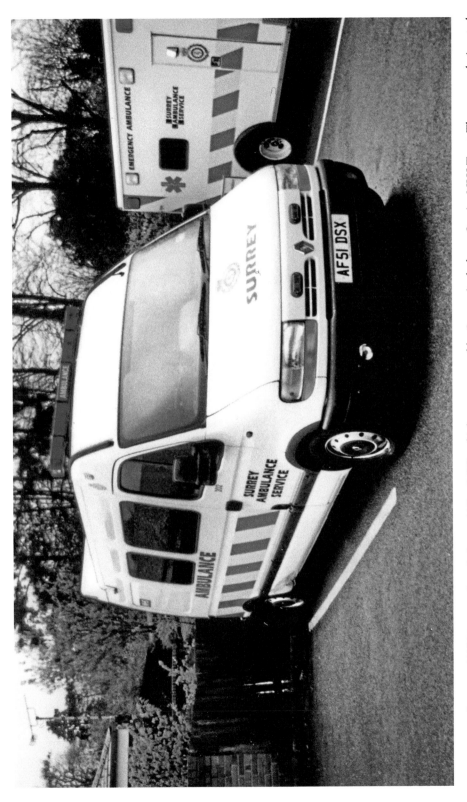

A 2001 Renault Master/ATT Papworth ambulance, (AF51 DSX), which was operated by Surrey Ambulance Service NHS Trust. These were designated as high-dependency units for rapid hospital-to-hospital transfer on blue lights.

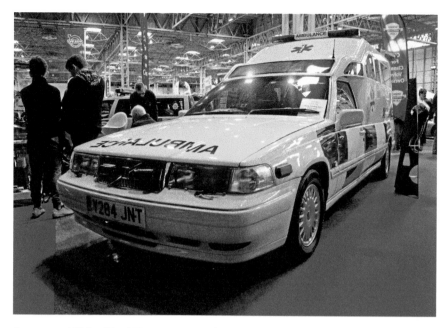

A preserved Volvo V90/Winman seen at the NEC Birmingham on 12 November 2016. This example, (Y283JNT), was originally operated by Shropshire Ambulance Service before being used for former Prime Minister Tony Blair as his ambulance. These car-derived conversions saw use in Shropshire, Wiltshire, Oxfordshire, and Northern Ireland. However, their operational life was relatively short-lived in the NHS.

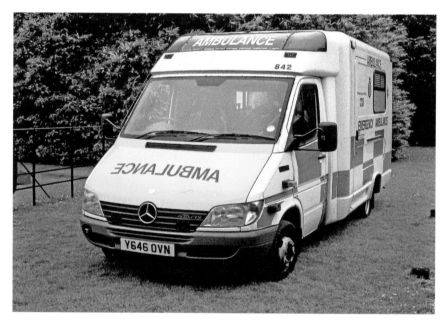

A 2001 Mercedes Benz 416CdI Sprinter/U.V.G 'Premia', (Y646OVN), operated by the North East Ambulance Service when seen on 19 May 2009, but had been new to the Tees, East and North Yorkshire Ambulance Service. These were a popular choice for many UK ambulance services.

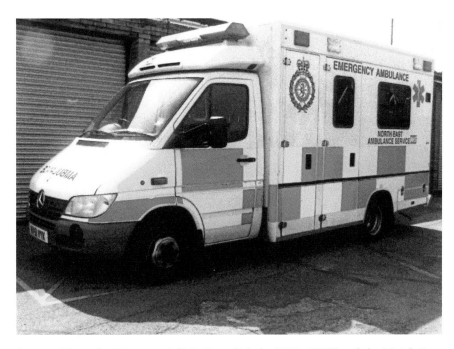

A 2001 Mercedes Benz 419CdI Sprinter/Jakab, (NV51VYK), of the North East Ambulance Service. This was purchased when NEAS had different boundaries to the 2006 reorganisation of ambulance services. This carries an all-over white colour, which has mainly gone on UK ambulances since 2003.

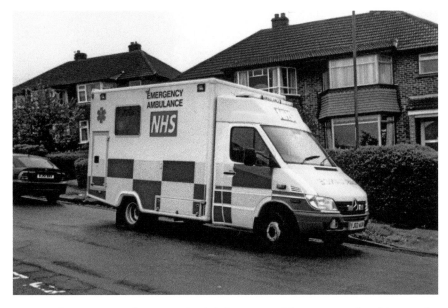

A Mercedes Benz 416CdI Sprinter/W.A.S. from 2003. These were ordered in 2002 by a consortium of northern ambulance services: Cumbria Ambulance Service, North East Ambulance Service, and Tees, East and North Yorkshire Ambulance Service. This particular example, (YJ03AUM), was a TENYAS ambulance. It was stolen and written off in January 2007.

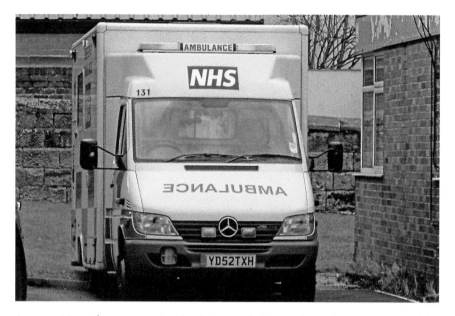

A 2002 Mercedes Benz 416 CdI/W.A.S. ambulance, (YD52TXH), operated by Yorkshire Ambulance Service NHS Trust as fleet number 131. This class was delayed in entering service (with the now-past Tees, East and North Yorkshire Ambulance Service) when it was found that the RICON lifts originally mounted under the rear doors were unsuitable for clearing speed bumps. Seen when in service at Whitby on 4 March 2009.

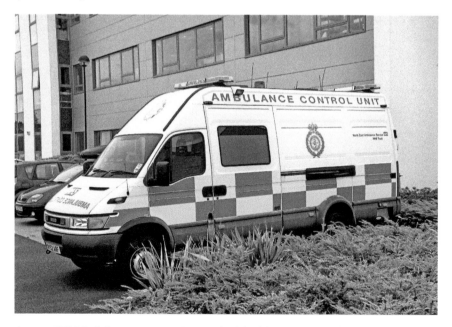

A 2002 IVECO daily van, (NY52ARF), which had been converted to a mobile control unit of North East Ambulance Service. This carried all service lettering, crown badge, blue and green lights, as well as having 'Ambulance Mobile Control' on the bonnet, along with the NHS logo. Photo taken 31 July 2008. This has now left the NHS.

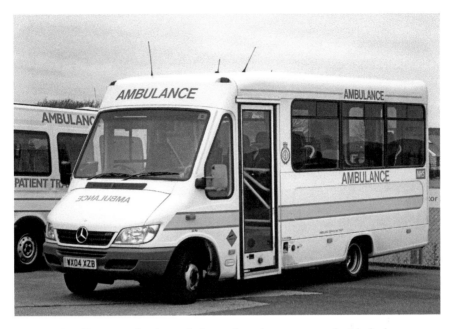

Most Patient Transport Service ambulances have been converted with the base van or minibus bodywork left unaltered. Having coach-built bodies is unusual to see. One such example that used specialised design was the Mercedes Benz 416CdI/UVModular 'Trekka' conversion. A former Tees, East and North Yorkshire Ambulance Service example, (WX04XZB) was one of a batch ordered in 2004.

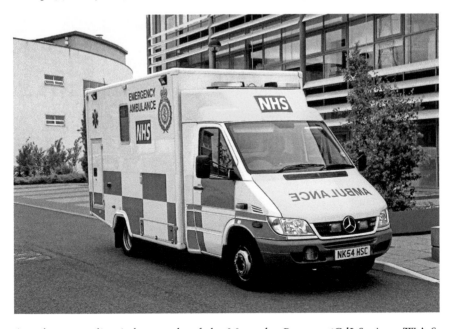

A rather more liveried example of the Mercedes Benz 416CdI Sprinter/W.A.S. Ambulances is this North East Ambulance Service example, (NK54HSC), seen in Newcastle-upon-Tyne. Many of these did not carry the NHS Ambulance Service lettering or crown badge.

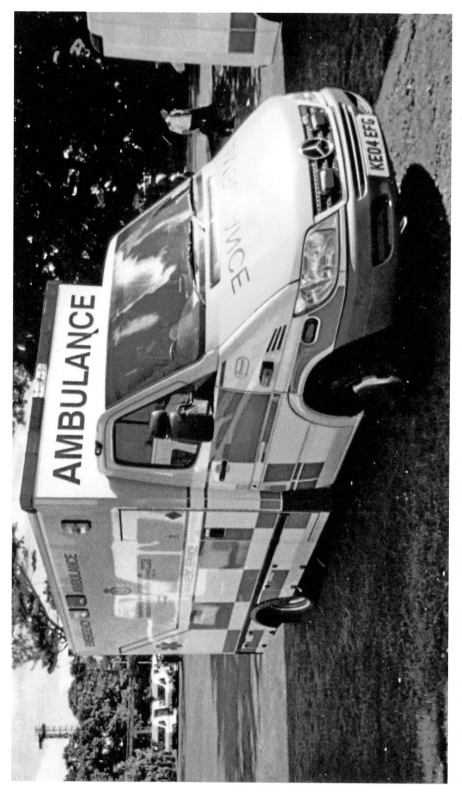

A 2004 Mercedes Benz 419CdI Sprinter/UVModular, (KE04EF), of the former Bedfordshire and Hertfordshire Ambulance Service NHS Trust. This ambulance was based in Bedfordshire and in 2006 became part of the East of England Ambulance Service.

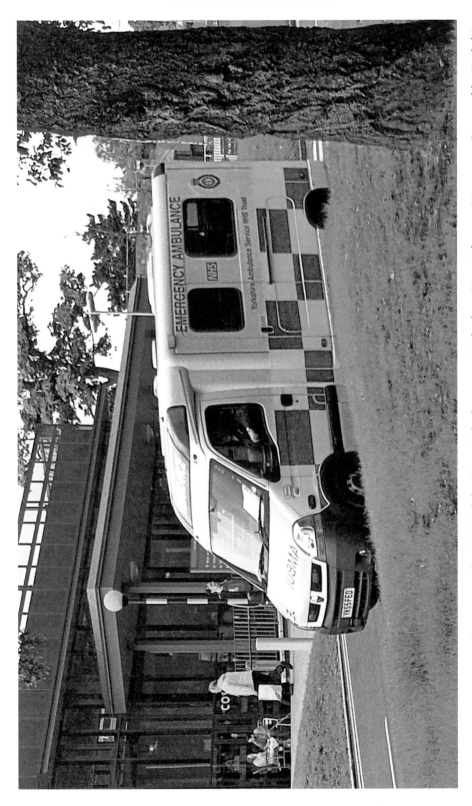

(YN55FED), a 2005 Renault Master with a UVModular 'Premia' body, seen at Rotherham Hospital on 15 May 2012. Operated by Yorkshire Ambulance Service, this was first used by South Yorkshire Ambulance Service.

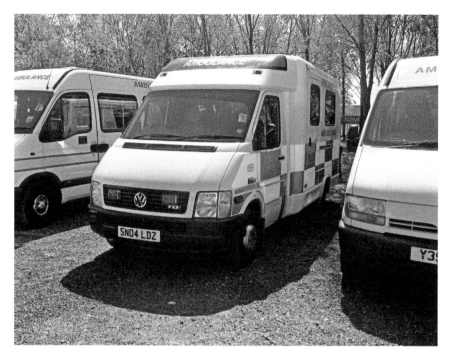

A large number of Scottish Ambulance Service vehicles were based on the VW LT40 with UVModular 'Premia' bodies. This example, (SN04LDZ), is seen just as it left the Scottish Ambulance Service.

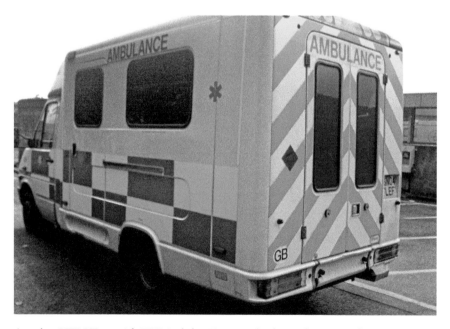

Another VW LT40 with UVModular 'Premia' bodies. This example, (SN04LEF), shows the low-profile doors that allowed a ramp to be used to load patients into the ambulance. This was at a time when rear-mounted stretcher lifts were becoming part of the design of ambulances.

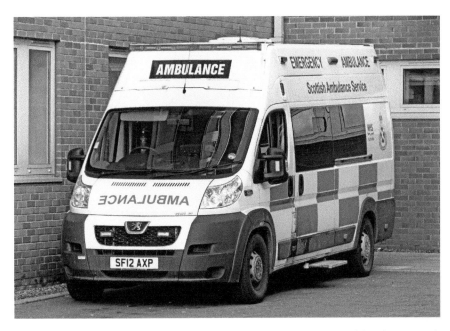

A 2012 Peugeot Boxer/Wilker conversion, (SF12AXP), operated by the Scottish
Ambulance Service. Seen at the Cumberland Infirmary, Carlisle. Scottish Ambulance
Service vehicles have never used the EEC117 yellow colour. Along with the
Mercedes Benz Sprinter, the Peugeot Boxers form a large part of the ambulance fleet
in Scotland.

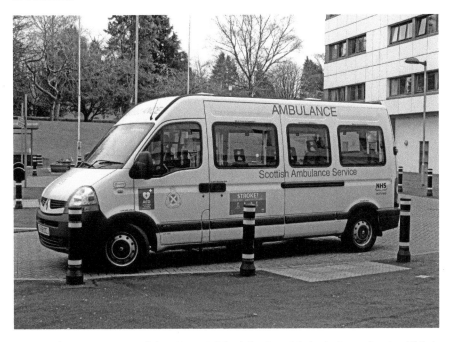

A Renault Master/UVModular, (SF58CCJ) of the Scottish Ambulance Service. This is
one of the service's Patient Transport Service ambulances for routine out-patient and
discharge work. It is seen at Dumfries hospital.

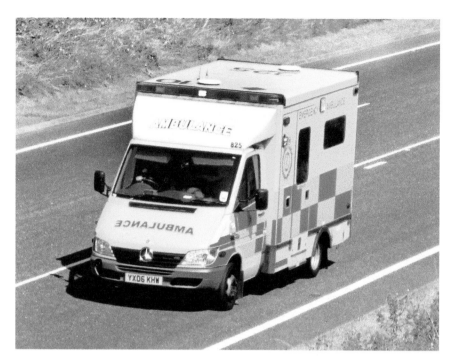

Another 2006 Mercedes Benz 416CdI/UVModular ambulance, (YX06KHW), operated by North East Ambulance Service NHS Trust. Fleet number/call sign 825 takes an emergency case along the A173 in Teesside.

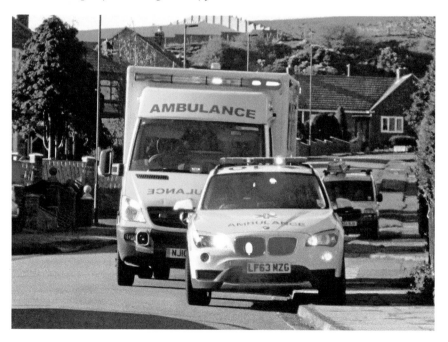

An emergency response is seen in charge of BMW X1/Safeguard SPV (LF63MZG) that would have arrived on scene before the Mercedes Benz 519CdI Sprinter/W.A.S. ambulance (NJ10DHK) – both of the North East Ambulance Service.

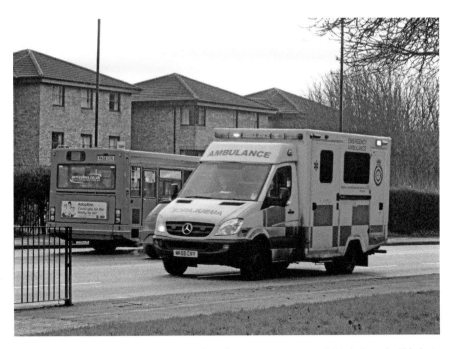

The North East Ambulance Service has for many years used W.A.S. to build their ambulances on Mercedes Benz chassis with the Sprinter 519CdI type being used. One example, (NK59CVY), is seen responding to an emergency call in Middlesbrough on 25 January 2014.

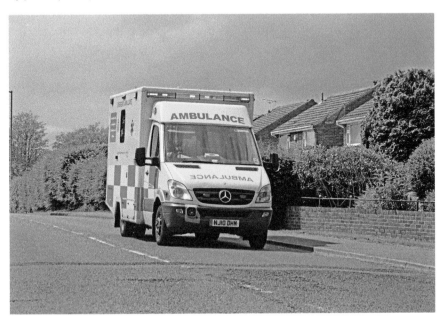

A 2010 Mercedes Benz 519 CdI Sprinter/W.A.S., (NJ10DHM), fleet number/call sign 291, of the North East Ambulance Service, seen on blue lights responding through Junction Road, Norton-on-Tees. This class have formed the backbone of the Teesside A&E fleet for many years.

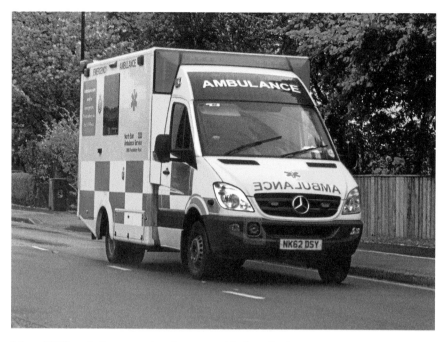

Many NHS ambulance services have put side-based adverts to encourage people to dial 999 for emergency situations only. From 2016, North East Ambulance Service began to apply these to its existing fleet. One is seen on this 2013 Mercedes Benz 519CdI Sprinter/W.A.S., (NK62DSY).

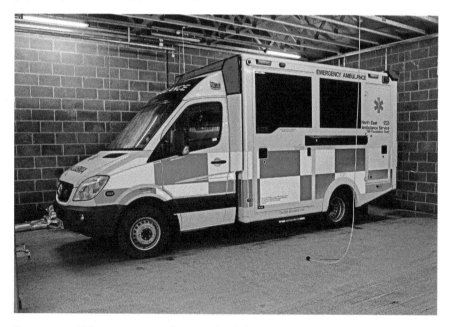

Seen on 12 February 2015 when newly delivered, and before the 999 posters were applied, was this North East Ambulance Service Mercedes Benz 519CdI Sprinter/W.A.S., (NK64TLN). The revised livery also denotes the service is an NHS Foundation Trust.

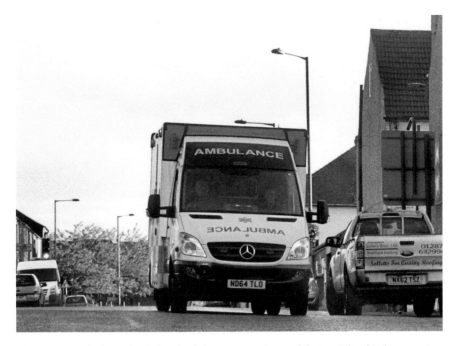

The WA.S. ambulance body has had three generations of design. The third generation changed from having a blue light bar over the cab to having a striking blue light design incorporated into the body design. The design is seen to good use in the North East Ambulance Service fleet as this example, (ND64TLO), shows.

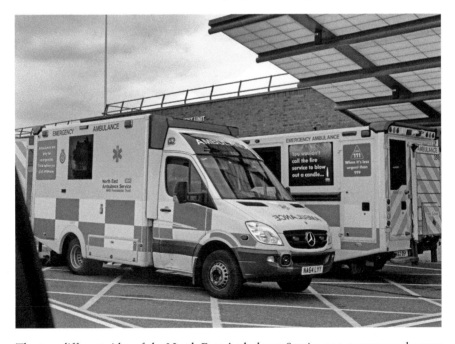

The two different sides of the North East Ambulance Service 999 posters can be seen with the offside red poster on (NA64LYY), while the nearside has details for the NHS non-emergency 111 service on (NK62DSY), 19 June 2016.

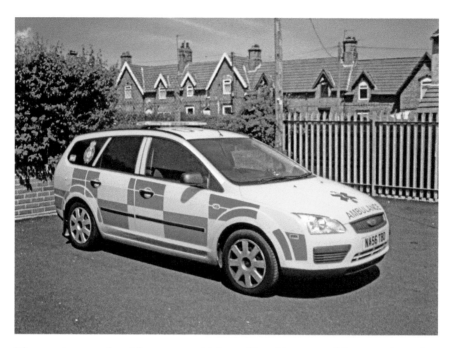

The growing use of rapid-response vehicles on Teesside occurred in 2006. A number of now-decommissioned Ford Focuses with UVModular conversions were purchased for use in this role. One of the first to arrive was this car, (NA56TBO), seen on 29 August 2007.

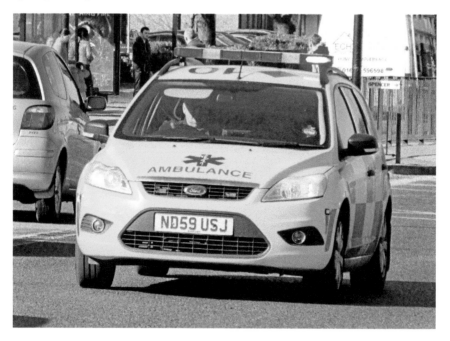

A photo of the older Ford Focus/UVModular rapid-response cars of the North East Ambulance Service showing (ND59USJ) when in service, responding to an emergency call on 12 March 2014.

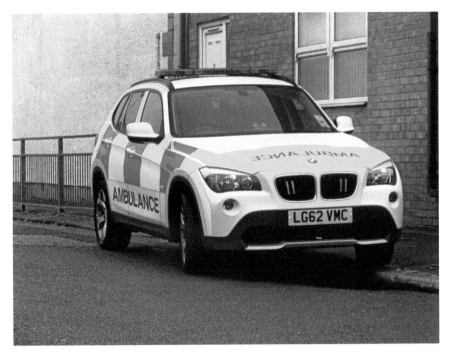

Another of the North East Ambulance Service BMW fleet, (LG62VMC) is seen in Bowburn, County Durham, in foggy conditions. This has a slightly different livery to the others in the fleet.

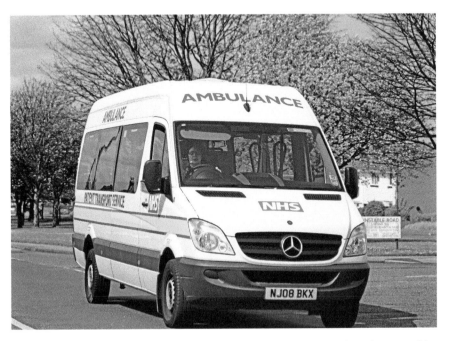

One of the larger Patient Transport Service ambulance fleet that have been used by North East Ambulance Service have been the Mercedes Benz 313CdI Sprinter with O&H conversion to PTS use. One of the fleet, (NJ08BKX), is seen 17 May 2016.

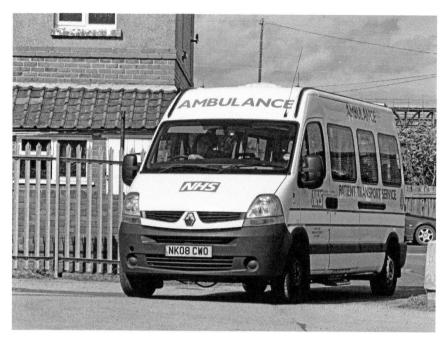

Another long-lived design for Patient Transport operations has been the Renault Master with O&H conversions, which have been a common sight around hospitals for many years. This North East Ambulance Service example, (NK08CWO), wearing the standardised livery, is typical of the class and was seen on 11 August 2014.

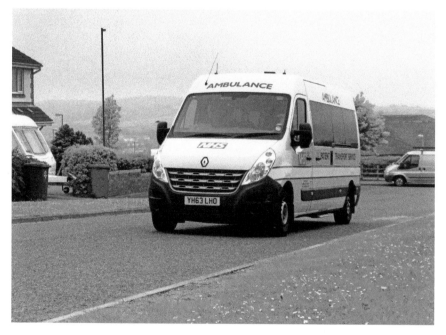

A 2013 Renault Master/O&H of the North East Ambulance Service, (YH63LHO). Operational for the Patient Transport Service, this ambulance is seen proceeding up Alford Road, Brotton, on 15 May 2016.

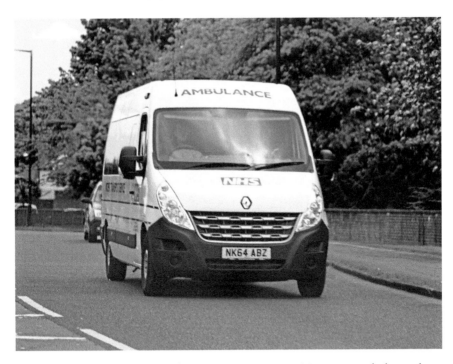

The newer generation of Renault Master/O&H Patient Transport ambulances have tinted saloon windows. The livery used remains unchanged in the North East fleet, as seen on one example: (NK64ABZ).

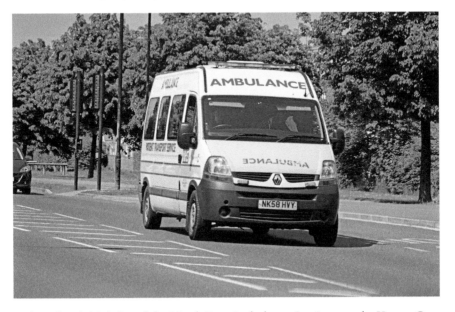

A short-lived third tier of the North East Ambulance Service was the Urgent Care transport fleet. These could be used for GP admissions to hospital. The Renault Master/O&H conversions had yellow warning bonnets and blue light bars added. Eventually they were used for Patient Transport stretcher case work and one of the class, (NK8HVY), is seen on such duty on 14 June 2016.

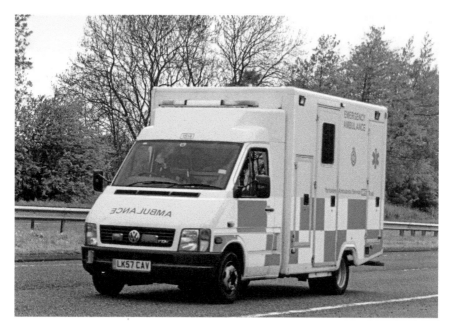

A 2007 VWLT40/W.A.S. of Yorkshire Ambulance Service. Yorkshire Ambulance Service operated a number of these London-registered VW LT40s in their fleet, which had older W.A.S. bodies that were refurbished by Wilker Ltd and mounted on the VW chassis. This example, (LK57CAV), fleet number 1514, is seen on the A171 near Guisborough on 9 September 2016.

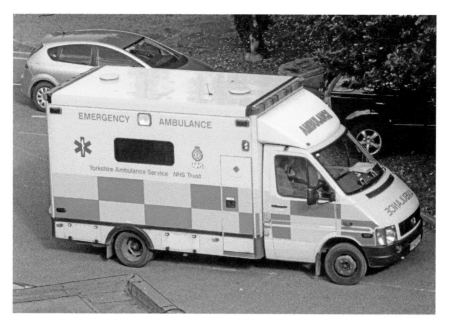

A former Yorkshire Ambulance Service ambulance is this VWLT40/UVModular, (YX07FPY), fleet number 166, seen when in service on 20 August 2014 at Whitby ambulance station. *Circa* 2007, Yorkshire Ambulance Service were using VW for some of their fleet.

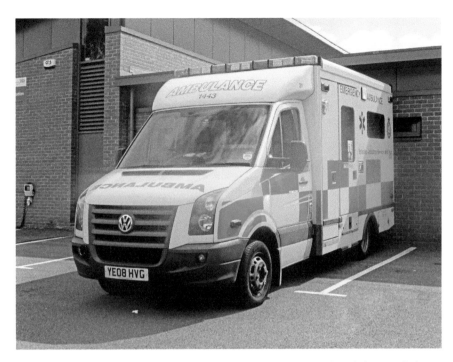

A VW Crafter/UVModular, (YEo8HVG), fleet number 1443, of Yorkshire Ambulance Service seen in Hull is one of a handful that were used by the service. A later fleet of VW crafters were purchased with different bodywork.

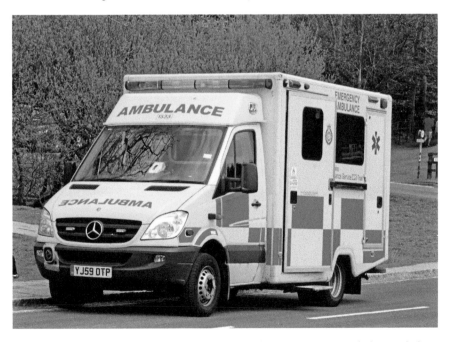

(YJ59OTP), a 2010 Mercedes Benz 519CdI Sprinter/W.A.S. of the Yorkshire Ambulance Service NHS Trust. One of the many in the standardised fleet, fleet number/call sign 1533 is seen on scene in Goathland, North Yorkshire.

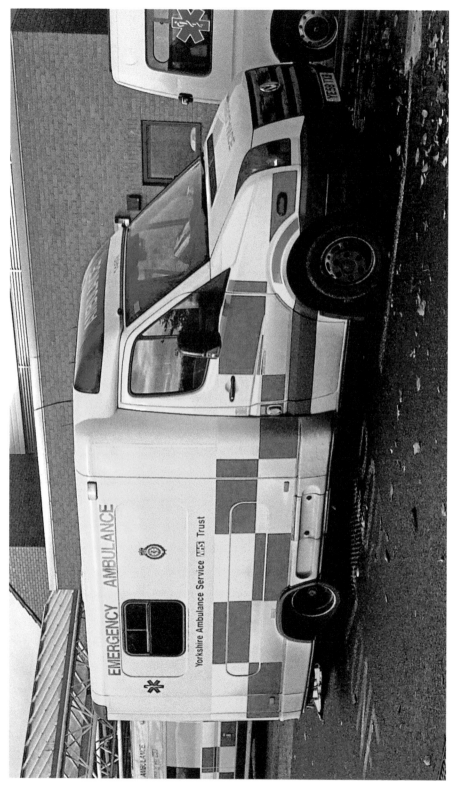

(YE58TXB), fleet number 1469, is a 2008 VW Crafter/UVModular 'Premia' frontliner of the Yorkshire Ambulance Service. The majority of the fleet were used in South Yorkshire around Sheffield.

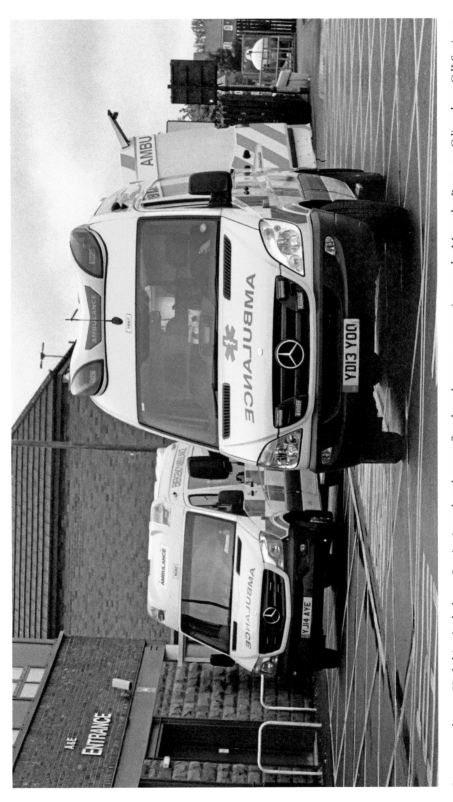

In 2013 and 2014 Yorkshire Ambulance Service introduced a new fleet based on van conversions to the Mercedes Benz 419Cdi and 519CdI Sprinter, rather than a modular body. On the left of the photo is the 2014 batch (YJ14AYE), fleet number 1692, which is a 519CdI Sprinter with Wilker Ltd. On the right is the 2013 arrival (YJ13YOO), fleet number 1667, with a 419CdI conversion by Cartwright.

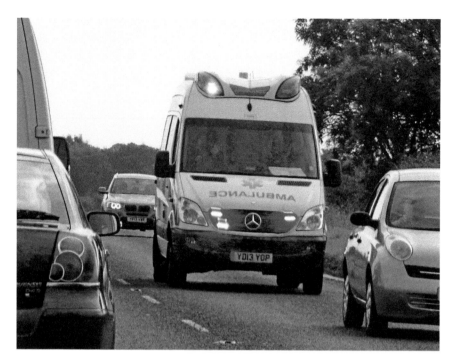

Showing the blue light cluster to good use is Yorkshire Ambulance Service Mercedes Benz 419CdI Sprinter/Cartwright (YO13 YOP), fleet number 1669, as it struggles to make headway to a 999 call on 20 September 2015.

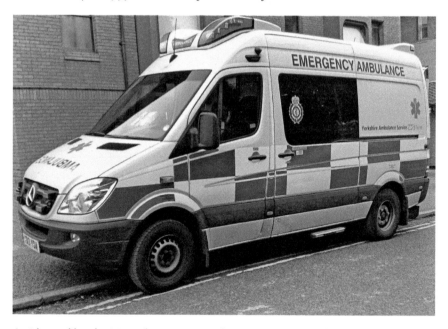

A side-profile of a Mercedes Benz 419CdI Sprinter/Cartwright, (YO13 YOA), fleet number 1664, shows how the conversion externally has not had major bodywork changes made from the base van. The conversion uses roof-mounted light pods for the blue lights.

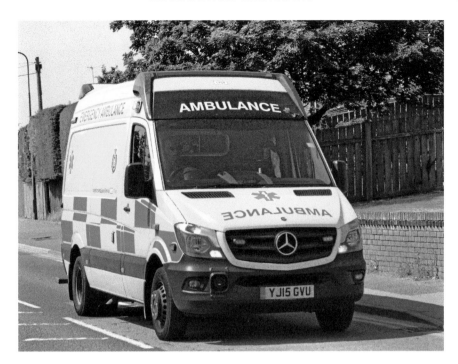

Another type of Mercedes Benz 519CdI Sprinter-based van conversion that had a delayed entry into service were a batch of W.A.S. converted ambulances. One of them, (YJ15GVU), fleet number 1754, passes through Bedale on 20 July 2016.

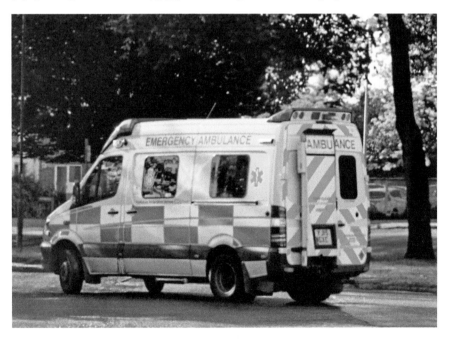

The back of Mercedes Benz 519CdI Sprinter/W.A.S. (YJ15GXC) shows the rear stretcher lift and saloon windows added in the conversion as it turns out onto a main road in Harrogate on 30 September 2016.

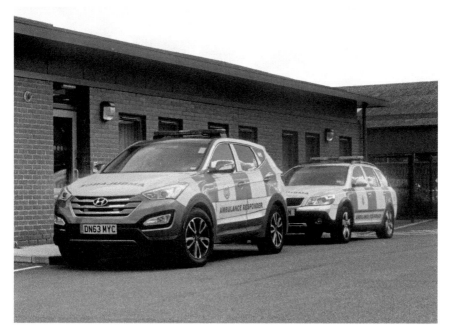

Two different types of rapid-response cars used by Yorkshire Ambulance Service are seen at Hull West ambulance station on 14 September 2014. (DN63MYC), fleet number 1398 – a 2014 Hyundi Santa Fe – stands in front of a 2013 Skoda Octavia Scout/Cartwright.

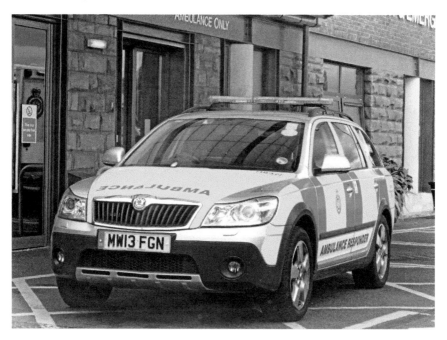

In 2013 Cartwright, as well as supplying ambulance conversions, also did a number of rapid-response car conversions to Skoda Octavia Scout 4x4 estates. Fleet number 1847, (MW13FGN), is seen outside an A&E department.

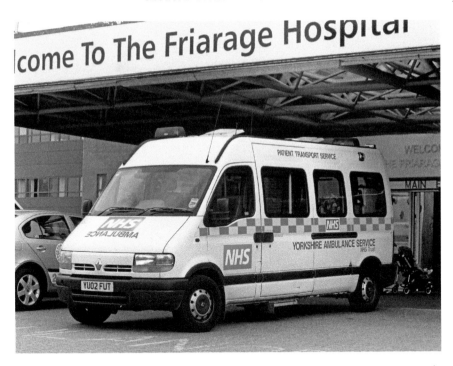

An ageing Renault Master Patient Transport ambulance, (YU02FUT), is seen 30 July 2014 at The Friarage Hospital, Northallerton. This was one of a number of Patient Transport Service ambulances that had small blue light beacons on the roof.

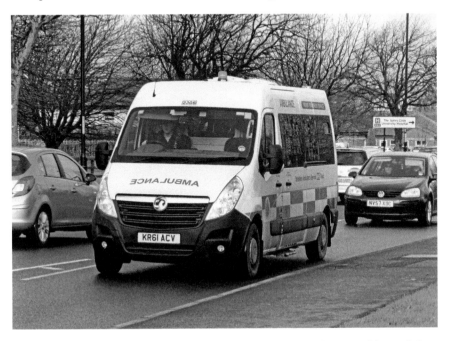

A small number of Vauxhall Movao/Wilker conversions have been used by Yorkshire ambulance service for Patient Transport Service work. One example, (KR61ACV), fleet number 2306, leaves a hospital on 29 January 2014.

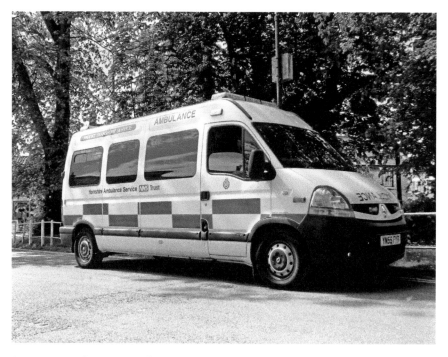

A 2009 Renault Master/Wilker of Yorkshire Ambulance Service, (YN59FYB). Patient Transport Service ambulance fleet number 2732 is seen in Thornton Le Dale, North Yorkshire, on 24 May 2015.

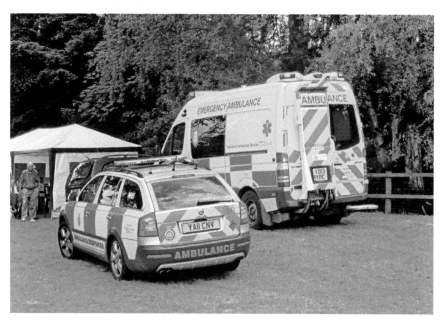

Two Yorkshire Ambulance Service frontline vehicles: (YA11CNV), a 2011 Skoda Octavia Scout rapid-response vehicle, fleet number 1921, next to (YD13YPC), a 2013 Mercedes Benz 419 CdI Sprinter/Cartwright ambulance, fleet number 1665 – seen at a call on 20 July 2014.

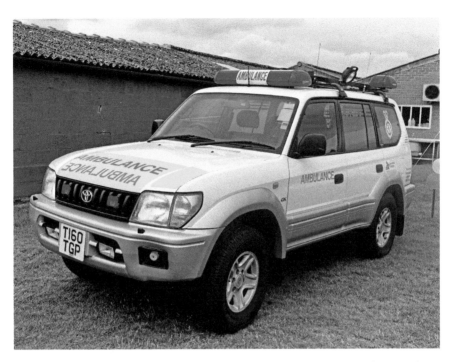

What is most likely the oldest vehicle in the fleet is this Toyota Landcruiser from 1999, (T160TGP), seen still in operation for Yorkshire Ambulance Service events team at Ripon on 24 July 2016.

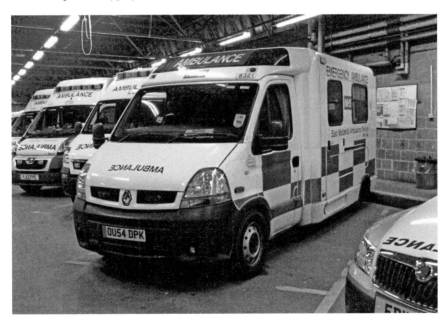

A 2004 Renault Master/UVModular 'Premia' ambulance of the East Midlands Ambulance Service, (OU54DPK). Allocated as call sign 8321, it is seen here on September 1 2012 at Kings Mill ambulance station in Sutton-In-Ashfield, Nottinghamshire. These have all been withdrawn from frontline operations.

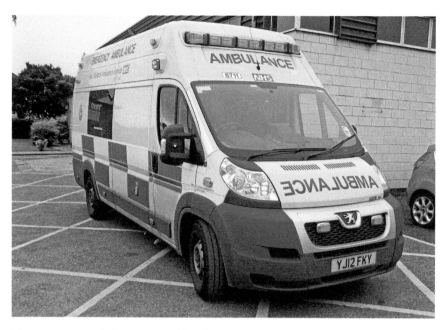

The mainstay of the East Midlands Ambulance Service fleet have been the Eurovan-based Peugeot Boxer and Fiat Ducato with O&H conversion to ambulances. The common example is of the Peugeot Boxer. One of the Skegness allocated ambulances, (YJ12FKY), fleet number 6711, is seen in October 2012, when new into service.

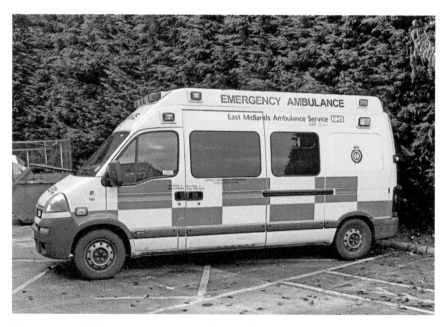

A 2010 Vauxhall Movano/O&H ambulance of East Midlands Ambulance Service, (YX59EJA), fleet number 8735, is seen at Alfreton, Derbyshire on 22 November 2012. Both the East Midlands Ambulance Service and West Midlands Ambulance Service used this type of ambulance.

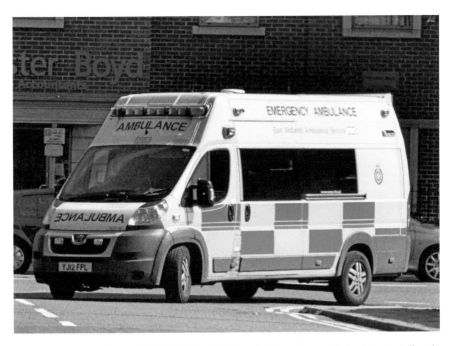

A 2012 Peugeot Boxer/O&H, (YJ12FPL), call sign 6920, of the East Midlands Ambulance Service is seen in Scunthorpe, North East Lincolnshire, on 11 September 2016. These conversions use the high roof van with ambulance conversion done on the interior, without major bodywork alterations externally.

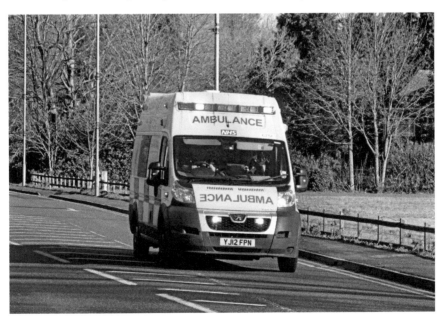

East Midlands Ambulance Service Peugeot Boxer/O&H ambulance, (YJ12FPN), fleet number 6712, seen on a blue light run on Sibsey Road in Boston, Lincolnshire, on 26 February 2014. The light bar has blue and white flashing lights in order to be more visible.

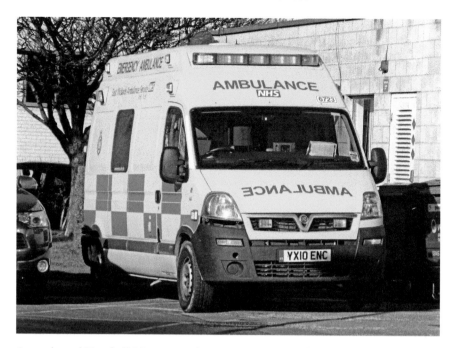

A number of Vauxhall Movano with O&H conversions have been operated by the East Midlands Ambulance Service. One example seen at Boston ambulance station in Lincolnshire is fleet number 6723, (YX10ENC), though these are slowly being phased out at time of writing.

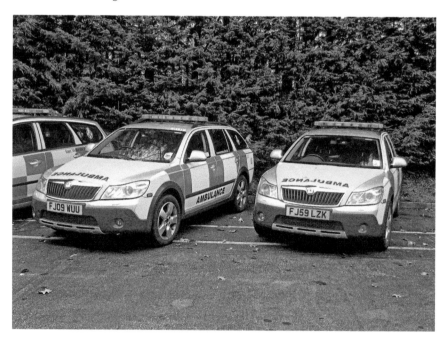

A pair of Skoda Octavia Scout/O&H rapid-response cars of the East Midlands Ambulance Service are seen awaiting their next turn of duty in Derbyshire. These were the cars that have been standardised over the six counties that EMAS cover.

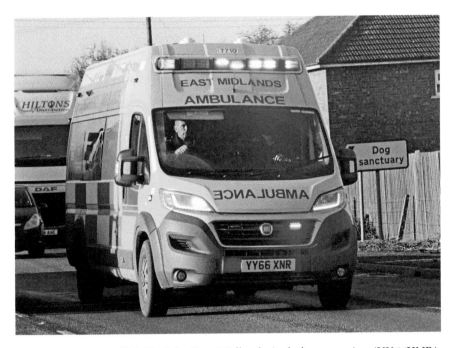

A 2016 Fiat Ducato/O&H of the East Midlands Ambulance service, (YY66XNR), fleet number 7710, runs to an emergency call past Sutterton, Lincolnshire, on the A17 on 4 January 2017. Since 2015, the wording of 'East Midlands' has been added to the over-cab lettering to distinguish the service operator.

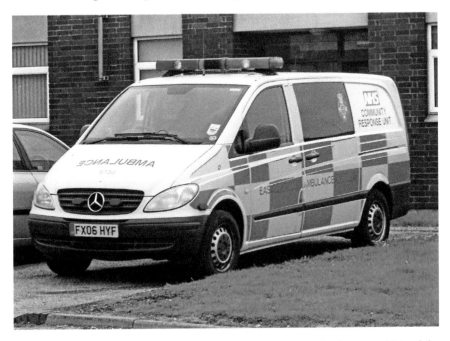

A now-decommissioned Mercedes Benz Vito/O&H Community Response Unit of the East Midlands Ambulance Service, (FX06HYF), seen at Skegness on 1 June 2012. These were used as Paramedic Response Units, mainly in Lincolnshire.

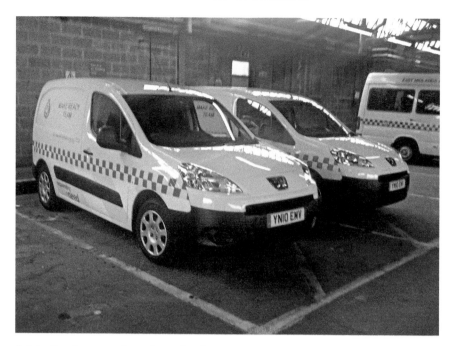

'Make Ready teams' have been developed since 2012 to prepare, stock, and check that ambulances are ready for duty before the crew book on duty. A number of vans have been put into service for their use, and these two Peugeot Experts are part of the East Midlands Ambulance Service team, seen at Kings Mill station in Nottinghamshire.

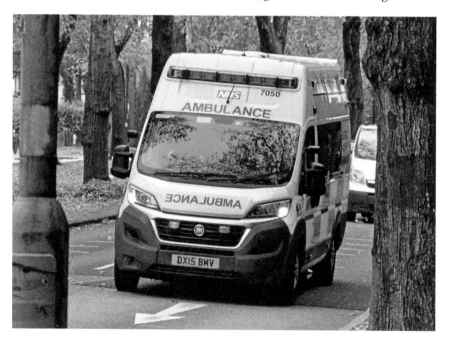

A Fiat Ducato with O&H conversion, (DX15BMV), fleet number 7050, of the West Midlands Ambulance Service. This is a driver training unit used by the ambulance service and matches the current West Midlands Ambulance Service fleet.

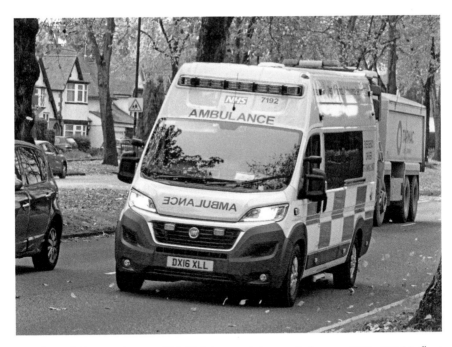

Another of the Fiat Ducato/O&H driver training ambulances, (DX16XLL), fleet number 7192, of the West Midlands Ambulance Service is seen in windy conditions on 26 October 2016. This has 'Emergency Driver Training Unit' lettered on the sides as well as the service name, and only has 'Ambulance' written on the front.

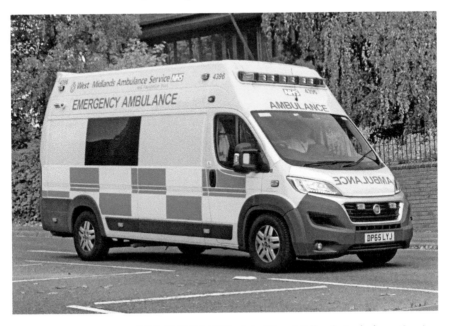

A 2016 Fiat Ducato Maxi/O&H (DP65LYJ) of the West Midlands Ambulance Service. Operational as fleet number 4396, this is seen near the University of Birmingham. With a lot of the side bodywork being free, the large reflective green-and-yellow 'Battenberg' squares can take a large portion of the sides.

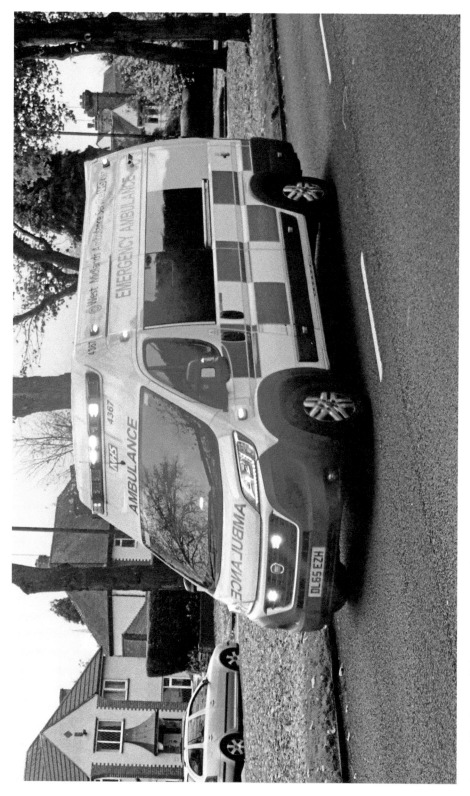

A 2015 Fiat Ducato/O&H (DL65EZH) of West Midlands Ambulance Service. Fleet number 4367 is seen on a blue light response on Bristol Road, Birmingham. This shows how the plethora of front and side lights make the ambulances as visible as possible while moving at high speeds.

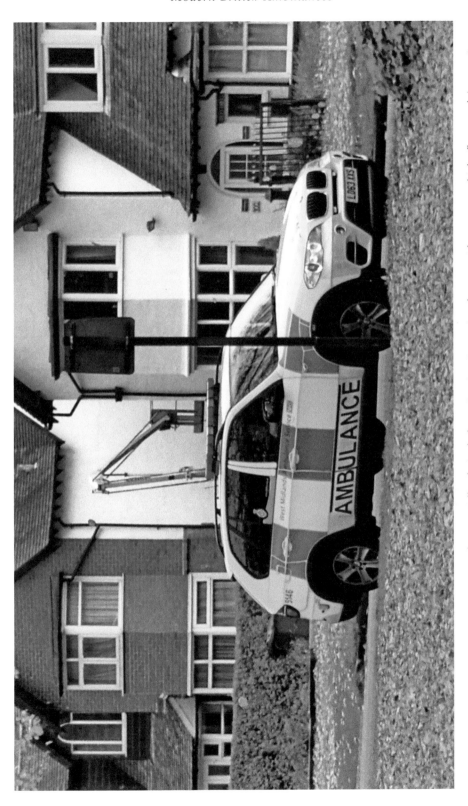

A 2014 BMW X5/Response SV (LD63XXS) of West Midlands Ambulance Service. Operational as a rapid-response vehicle, fleet number 5146 is seen on the A38 in Birmingham. The BMW X series have been used as a response car by several ambulance services.

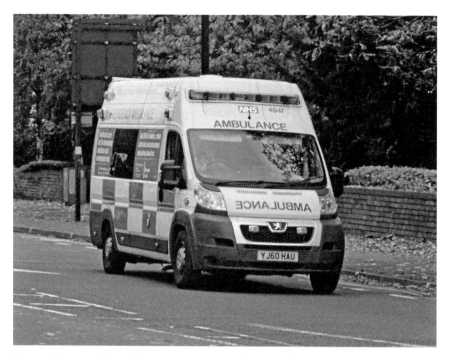

A 2010 Peugeot Boxer/O&H, (YJ60HAU), fleet number 4047, is one of the older Eurovan conversions for West Midlands Ambulance Service. It is seen with a side advert for 999 choices.

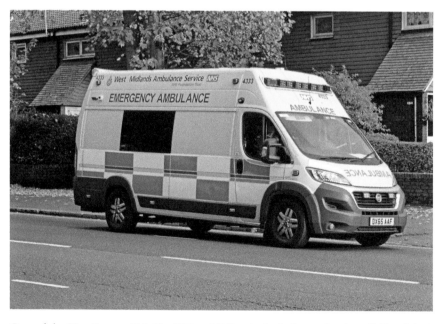

One of the Fiat Ducato/O&H of West Midlands Ambulance Service, (DX65AAF), fleet number 4333, from the 2015 fleet is seen near The Priory Hospital, Birmingham, showing the placing of side-lettering favouring the area near the roof to avoid being obscured in traffic.

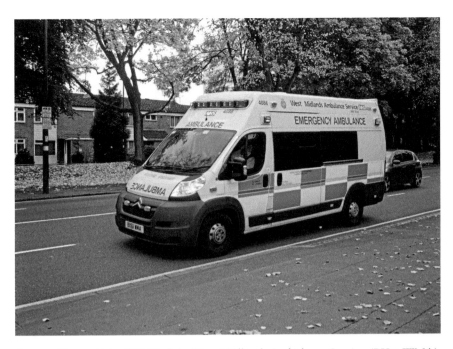

A 2012 Citroen Relay/O&H of the West Midlands Ambulance Service, (BX61WMA). Operational as fleet number 4086 in Birmingham, it is seen in the Edgbaston area of the city. At one time WMAS had a large number of Citroen ambulances on frontline work.

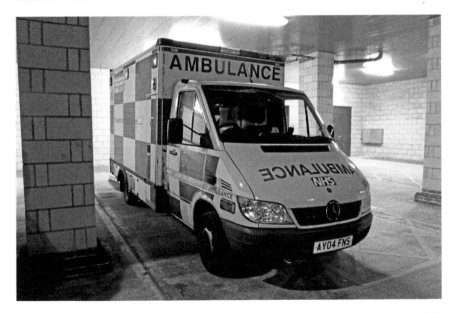

A former East of England Ambulance Service frontliner, number 974 is seen while in service on 22 February 2013 at Peterborough City Hospital. New to the former East Anglia Ambulance Service, this Mercedes Benz 416CdI Sprinter (AY04FNS) had a body constructed by UVModular. The design did not have an aerodynamic over-cab fairing.

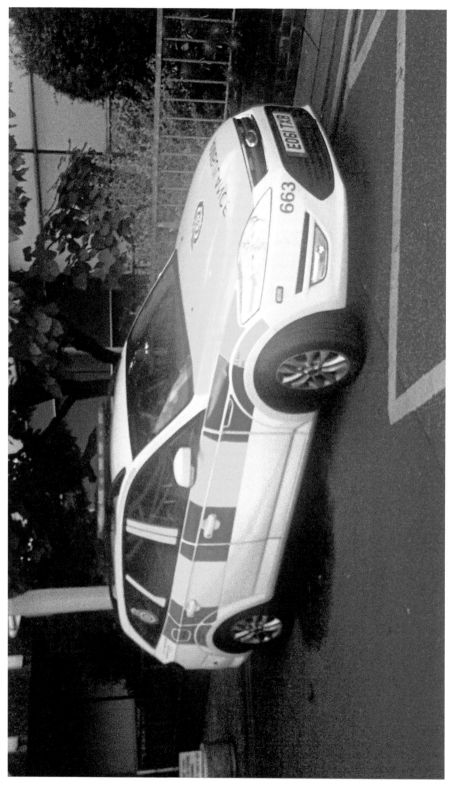

A Ford Mondeo/Wilker rapid-response car of the East of England Ambulance Service, (EO61TXB), fleet number 663, is seen at Addenbrookes Hospital, Cambridge, on 30 August 2012.

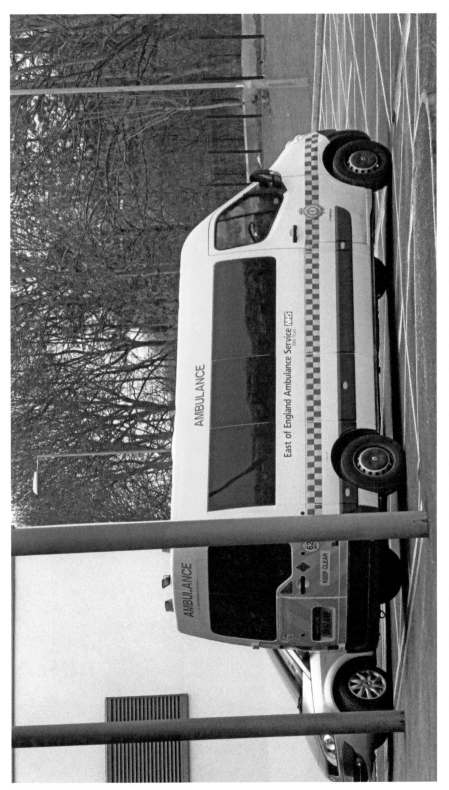

A 2011 Renault Master/Wilker ambulance, (DK61ANR), of the East of England Ambulance Service NHS Trust is seen at Peterborough City Hospital on 13 February 2013. This is one of the service's Patient Transport fleet. The ambulance has been governed to 62 mph and this is displayed on the rear door markings.

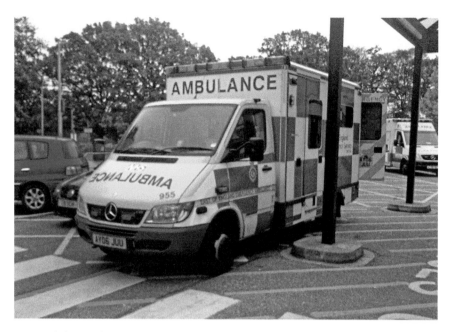

Seen while on duty at Queen Elizabeth Hospital, Kings Lynn, Norfolk, on October 19 2012 is (AU06JUU). A 2006 UVModular-bodied Mercedes Benz 416CdI Sprinter of the East of England Ambulance Service, fleet number 955 is now decommissioned but was based at Kings Lynn in service. The ambulance has the old East Anglia Ambulance Service all-over 'Battenberg' marking.

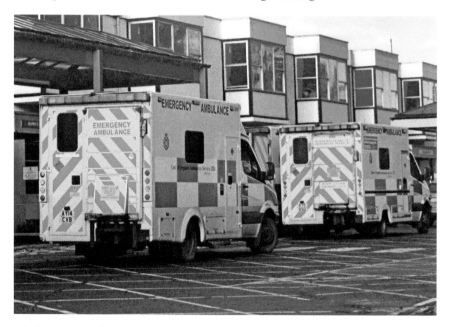

The back view of two Mercedes Benz 519CdI Sprinter/W.A.S. of East of England Ambulance Service showing the subtle changes over time. The newer ambulance from 2014, (AY14CVB), fleet number 899, is limited to 70 mph while the older 2011 ambulance, (AY11ASO), fleet number 252, is unrestricted.

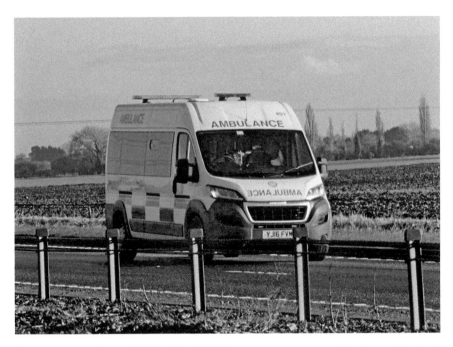

A 2016 Peugeot Boxer/O&H, (YJ16FVM), fleet number 401, of the East of England Ambulance Service. This is part of the service's Patient Transport fleet. There are blue light bars fitted, indicating the use of Urgent Care work can be done. This ambulance is seen on the A47 near Wisbeach, Cambridgeshire, on 5 January 2017.

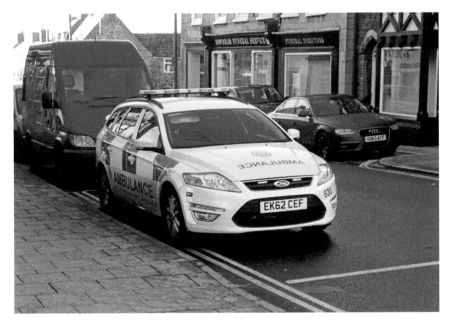

A Ford Mondeo/Wilker rapid-response vehicle of the East of England Ambulance Service, (EK62CEF), number 630. This is seen in Downham Market, Norfolk, on 5 January 2017. Unlike the ambulances of East of England, the response cars have white bodywork.

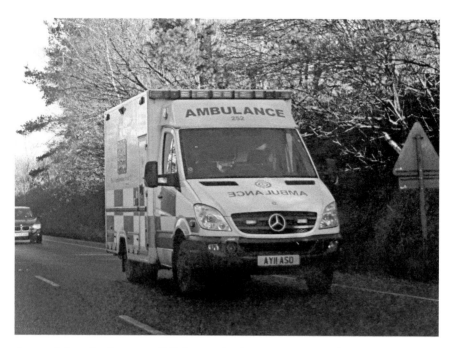

A 2011 Mercedes Benz 519 CdI Sprinter/W.A.S., (AY11ASO), fleet number 252, of the East of England Ambulance Service, is seen on the A149 near South Wooton, Norfolk. These W.A.S. bodies differ from the more commonly used design, and form the mainstay of the ambulance fleet for the service.

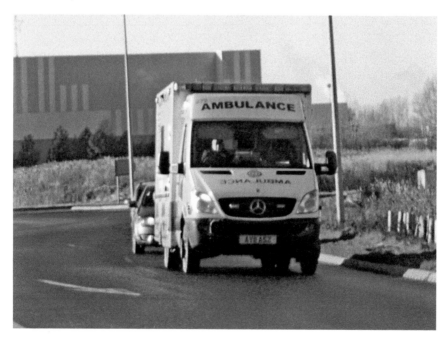

A 2011 Mercedes Benz 519 CdI Sprinter/W.A.S., (AY11ASZ), fleet number 272, of the East of England Ambulance Service is seen on the A149 near Kings Lynn, Norfolk. This is another of the standardised ambulances.

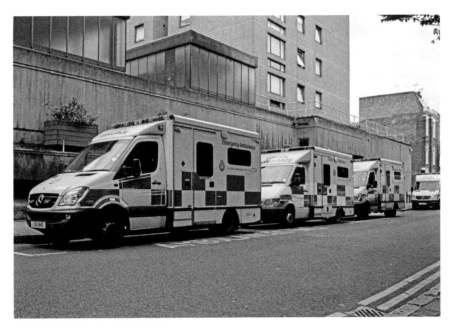

Four Mercedes Benz ambulances seen outside London Ambulance Service headquarters on Pearlman Street, Waterloo. (LC61BHO), fleet number 6888 – a MacNeillie-bodied ambulance – is in front, followed by (LJ53BVW), 2003 UVModular-bodied fleet number 6899, with (LJ09OMT), 2009 UVModular-bodied fleet number 7693, ending the first three. In the rear is (LJ58OJW), 2008 UVModular-bodied fleet number 7596.

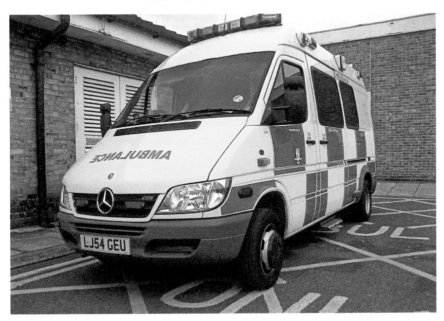

An ex-London Ambulance Service Urgent Care-tier ambulance is (LJ54GEU), a 2004 Mercedes Benz 416CdI Sprinter/MacNeillie, seen when in use on NHS support work on 14 May 2013 at Grantham hospital, Lincolnshire. Many of these ambulances are in use with private providers.

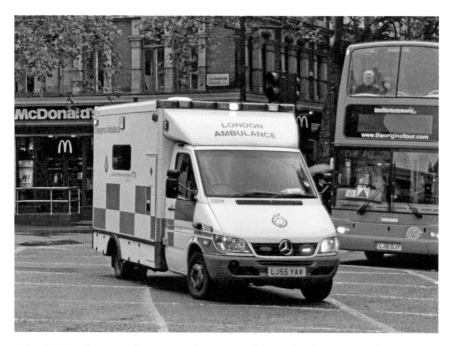

(LJ55YAV), fleet number 7225, is a 2005 Mercedes Benz 416CdI Sprinter/
UVModular of the London Ambulance Service. It is seen running on blue lights over
Cambridge Circus at the junction of Shaftsbury Avenue and Charing Cross Road in
Holborn, London.

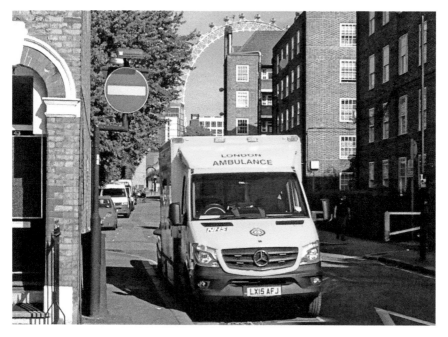

With the iconic London Eye dominating the background, London Ambulance Service
Mercedes Benz 519Cdi Sprinter/Mac Nellie (LX15AFJ), fleet number 8212, is seen
parked up in the sunshine on 28 June 2016.

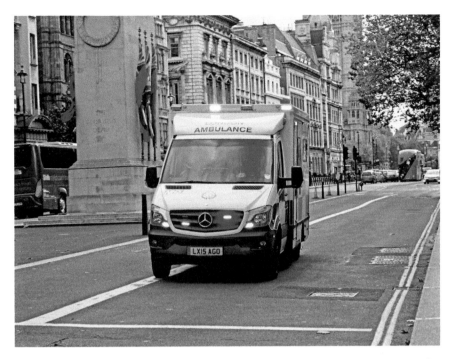

An emergency call on 16 October 2016 sees London Ambulance Service Mercedes Benz 519CdI Sprinter/MacNeillie (LX15AGO), fleet number 8199, run on blue lights and sirens past the cenotaph en route to the scene of the call.

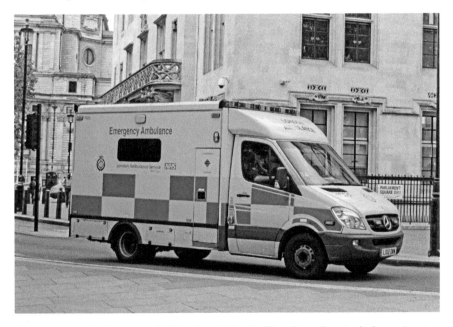

A 2012 Mercedes Benz 519CdI Sprinter/MacNeillie of London Ambulance Service, (LX12DWW), fleet number 7926, is seen passing through Parliament Square in Westminster on 29 June 2016. The Merseyside-based company MacNeillie have been providing the capital's ambulance fleet since 2004.

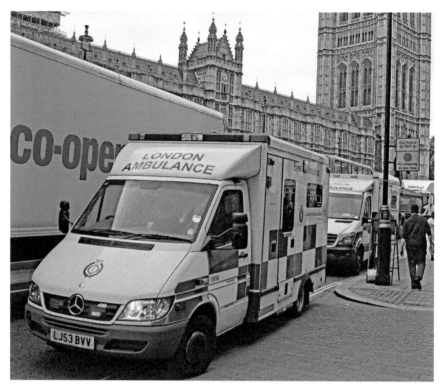

A pair of London Ambulances seen outside the Palace of Westminster. (LJ53BVV), a 2003 Mercedes Benz 416CdI Sprinter/UVModular, fleet number 6898, is marked as an event ambulance. Parked behind it is (LX15AHO), 2015 Mercedes Benz 519CdI Sprinter/MacNeillie, fleet number 8180, from the LAS duty emergency fleet.

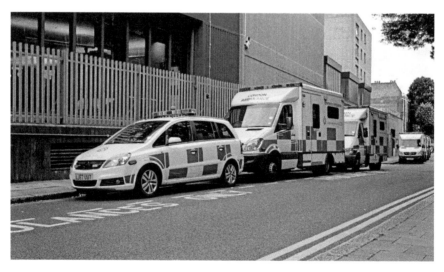

A London Ambulance Service trio seen on Pearlman Street, Waterloo. (LJ57UUT), a 2007 Vauxhall Zafira rapid-response car, fleet number 7437, is at the front. Behind it is a MacNeillie-bodied Mercedes Benz 519Cdi Sprinter, fleet number 7600, and last is an unidentified Mercedes Benz 416CdI Sprinter/UVModular.

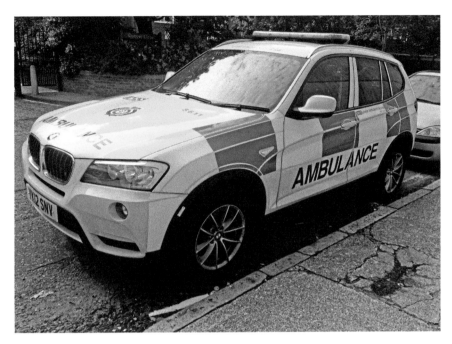

A BMW X5 rapid-response vehicle of London Ambulance Service, (YK12SNV), fleet number 5611. These are used by paramedic officers of the service. Along with the BMW, the London Ambulance Service also uses Skoda Octavias, which replaced older Vauxhall Zafira cars.

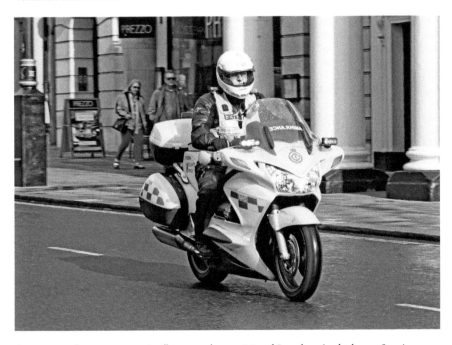

A motorcycle response unit, fleet number 7588, of London Ambulance Service seen on an emergency response on 16 October 2016. The motorbikes can negotiate the traffic far easier than cars and van-derived ambulances.

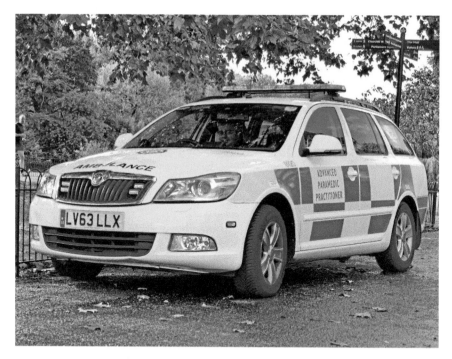

A Skoda Octavia Scout response car used by advanced paramedic practitioners of London Ambulance Service. This example, (LV63LLX), fleet number 8120, is seen on standby in Green Park, London. (Stuart McKenzie)

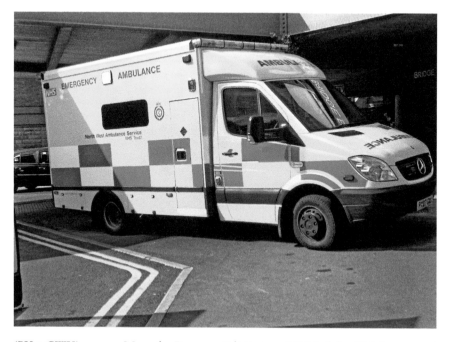

(PX07GWX), a 2007 Mercedes Benz 519CdI Sprinter/UVModular. This is operated by the North West Ambulance Service NHS Trust and was based in Cumbria. Some of these have recently been refurbished by Wilker Limited to extend their service life.

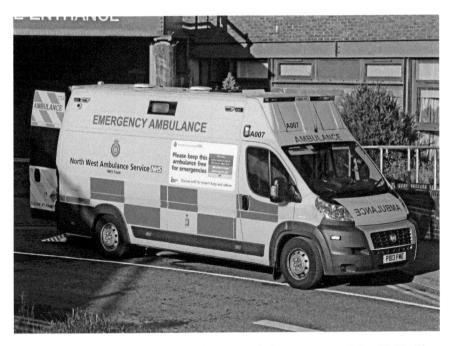

A 2013 Fiat Ducato/Wilker of North West Ambulance Service, (PO13FME). Fleet number A007 is one of a number of van conversions operated by NWAS. It also has an advert on the side urging the public to keep the ambulance service for emergencies only when seen on 2 February 2014.

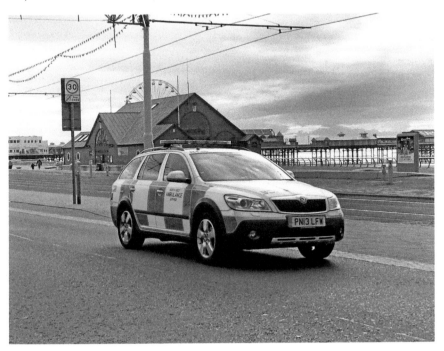

A 2013 Skoda Octavia/MacNeillie (PN13LFW) rapid-response vehicle of North West Ambulance Service. Fleet number R136 is seen in Blackpool on 18 February 2015.

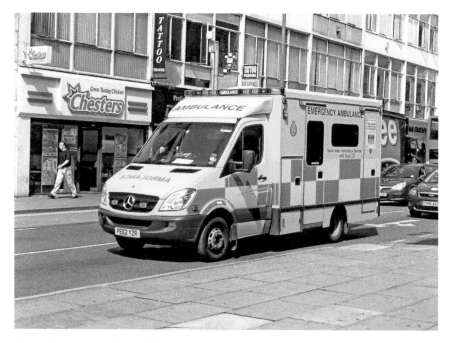

On 16 June 2014, PE62YZR 2012 Mercedes Benz 519 CdI Sprinter/MacNeillie of North West Ambulance Service (NWAS) is seen passing along Lime Street, Liverpool. The ambulance carries a sign advising the 999 number being for emergencies only. (Stuart McKenzie)

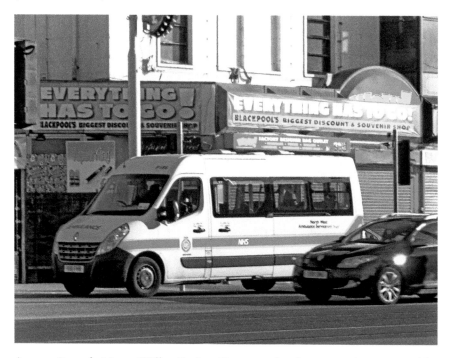

A 2011 Renault Master/Wilker Patient Transport Service conversion operated by North West Ambulance Service, (PO61FHR), number P1816, is seen in Blackpool.

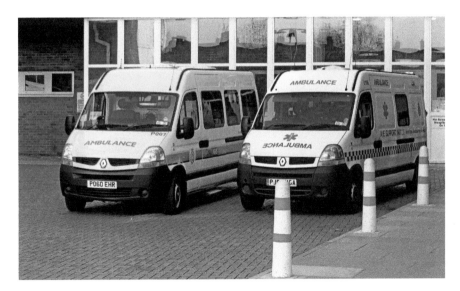

Two Renault Master/O&H conversions seen side by side on 29 January 2014. Left, (PO60EHR), number P007, is a Patient Transport Service ambulance. On the right, (PJ54UGA), fleet number U101, is from the A&E support tier.

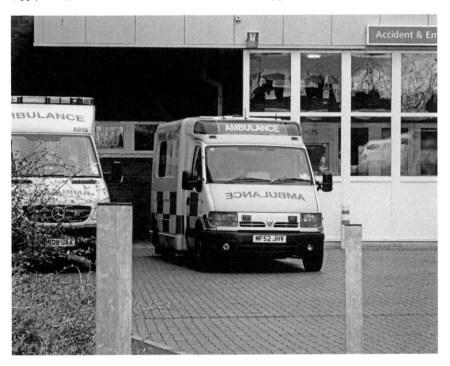

An old frontline ambulance, possibly a former Greater Manchester Ambulance Service ambulance, (MF52JHV) – a Renault Master/UVG 'Premia' – is seen at Carlisle in 2014 as part of the North West Ambulance Service fleet. The 'Premia' body was made initially by UVG and by UVModular when UVG merged. Following UVModular being liquidated in 2009 Wilker produced the body, mainly on Ford Transits, for the Scottish Ambulance Service.

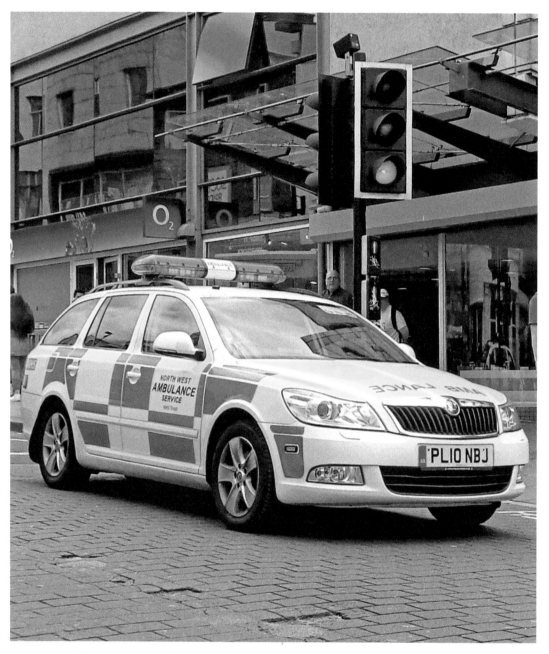

A Skoda Octavia with MacNeillie conversion of North West Ambulance Service, (PL10NBJ), fleet number R631, is seen in Liverpool leaving the scene of a call. This conversion used an oversized light bar mounted on the roof which is different to the LED-style blue light bars normally used.

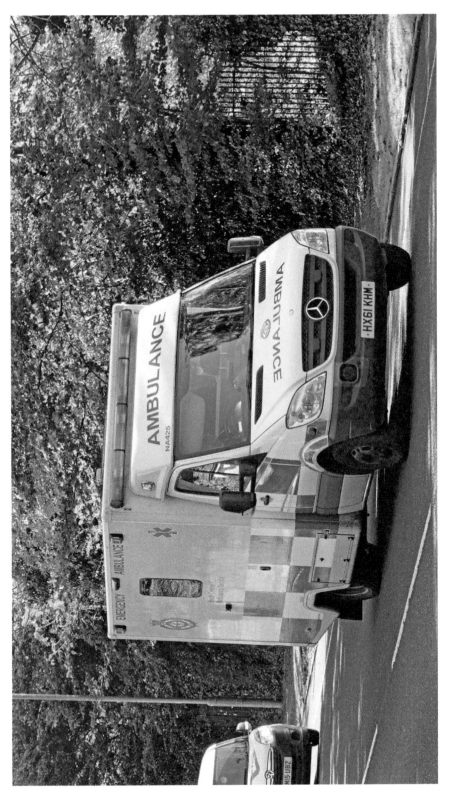

A 2011 Mercedes Benz 519CdI Sprinter/W.A.S., (HX61KHM), of South Central Ambulance service. Fleet number NA245 is seen passing through Heddington, Oxford, on 11 October 2016. The South Central ambulance fleet have used a white front on their yellow bodied ambulances; a reversal of when yellow was used on the front of white ambulances.

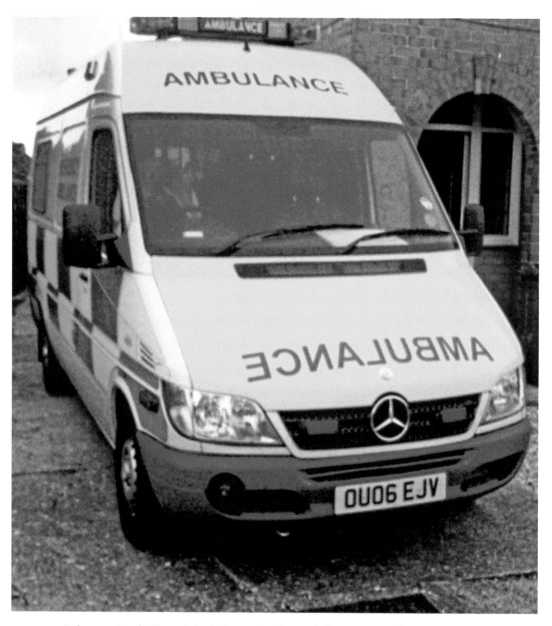

A former South Central Ambulance Service ambulance, Mercedes Benz 416CdI Sprinter/Wilker (OU06EJV), former fleet number 203, was based in Oxfordshire. This was a conversion on the basic van with an interior conversion being the main alteration.

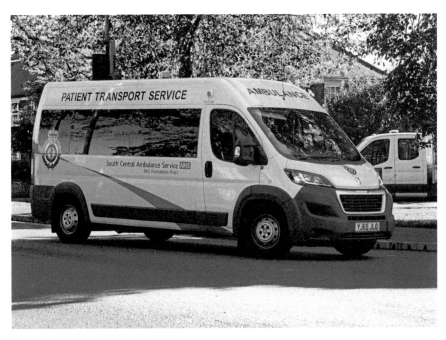

A 2015 Peugeot Boxer/O&H Patient Transport Service ambulance, (YJ65JLO) of South Central Ambulance Service. Fleet number NP338 is seen wearing a different take on the green-and-yellow livery as it passes through Oxford.

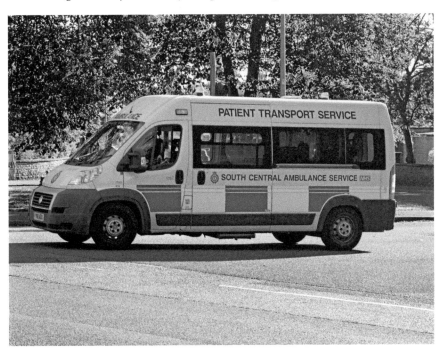

A 2011 Fiat Ducato/O&H, (YN11ADX), of South Central Ambulance Service's Patient Transport Service. Fleet number NP991 is seen in Oxford en route to the city's John Radcliffe Hospital.

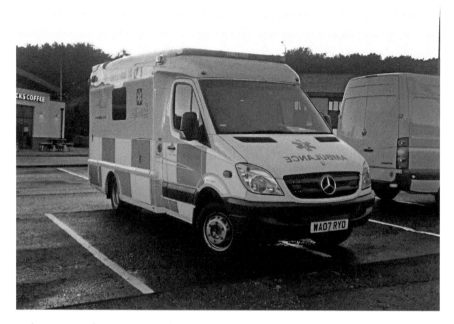

A former South Western Ambulance Service ambulance, (WA07RYO) – a 2007 Mercedes Benz 519CdI Sprinter/ATT Papworth – is seen operational with Medics UK. Many of these have now left service in the NHS and are finding a second life with private providers.

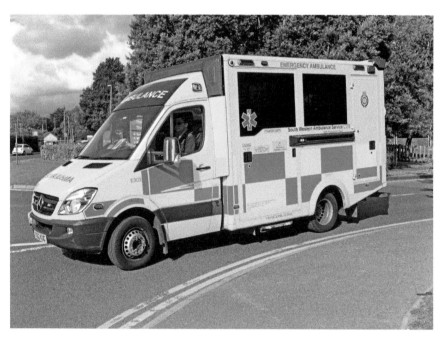

A 2013 Mercedes Benz 519CdI Sprinter/W.A.S. Third generation (VX62KUG) of South Western Ambulance Service, call sign E302, is seen in Gloucester – one of the service's fleet of emergency ambulances.

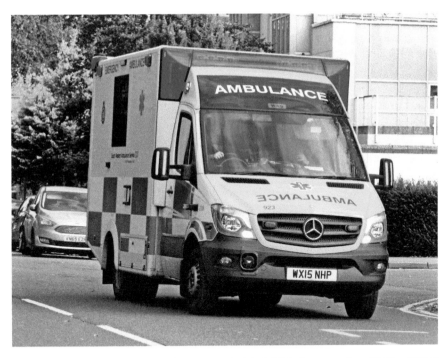

A 2015 Mercedes Benz 519CdI Sprinter/W.A.S. Third generation (WX15NHP) of South Western Ambulance Service, call sign E516/fleet number 923, is seen in Cheltenham. This is one of the newer generation of ambulances to enter service.

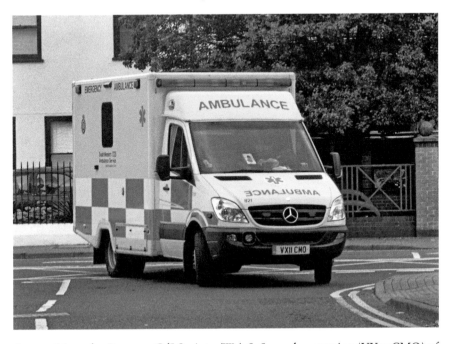

A 2011 Mercedes Benz 519CdI Sprinter/W.A.S. Second generation (VX11CMO) of South Western Ambulance service NHS Trust, fleet number 821/call sign E101, is seen in Gloucester on 12 October 2016.

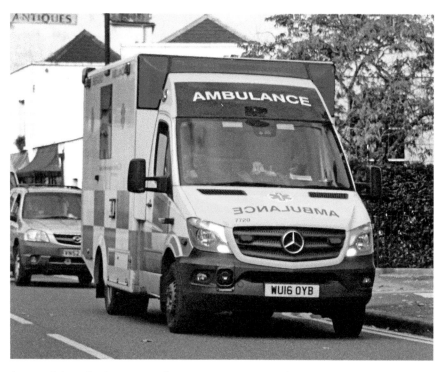

A 2016 Mercedes Benz 519CdI Sprinter/W.A.S. Third generation (WU16OYB) of South Western Ambulance Service, fleet number 7720, is seen in Cheltenham.

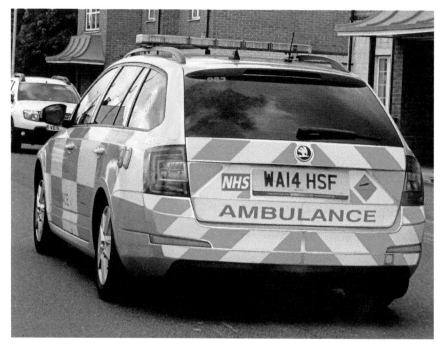

A Skoda Octavia rapid-response car, (WA14HSF) of South Western Ambulance Service, fleet number 983, is wearing a large 'Battenberg' green-and-yellow livery.

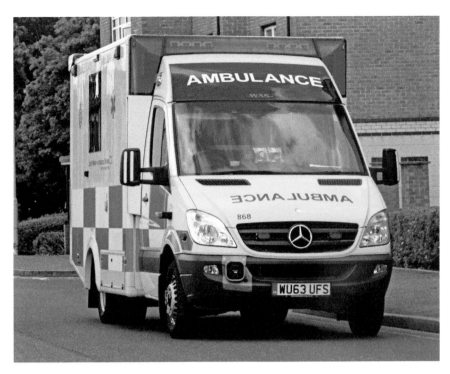

A 2013 Mercedes Benz 519CdI Sprinter/W.A.S. Third generation (WU63UFS) of South Western Ambulance Service, fleet number 868 is seen in Gloucester.

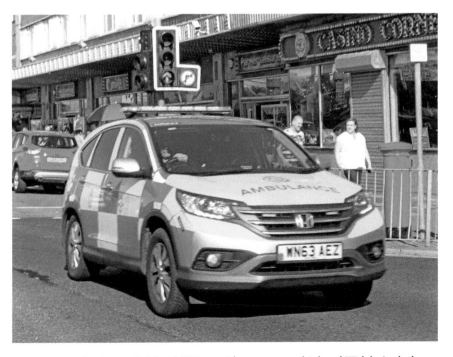

A 2013 Honda CR-V, (WN63AEZ); rapid-response vehicle of Welsh Ambulance Service. Fleet number NR002 is seen in Bangor on 27 September 2016.

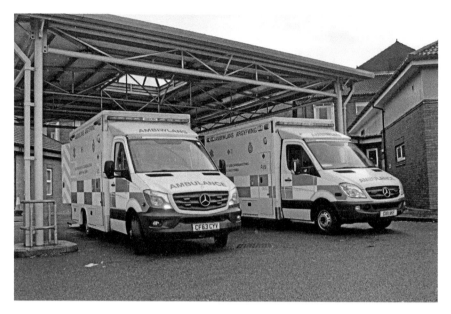

Two Mercedes Benz 519CdI Sprinter with Wilker conversions of the Welsh Ambulance Service NHS Trust seen on 9 November 2016 at Wrexham. Number NA263, (CF63CYV), is from 2013 while number NA300, (CX11AKF), is from 2011. These have the dual Welsh/English lettering on the sides with the nearside reading 'Welsh Ambulance Service NHS Trust', while on the offside the Welsh lettering 'Ymodreaudaeth Gig gwasanaethau ambiwlans Cymru' can be seen.

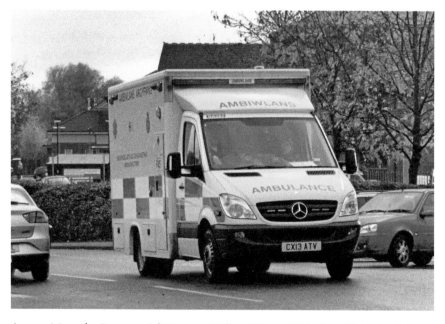

A 2013 Mercedes Benz 519CdI Sprinter/Wilker (CX13ATV) of the Welsh Ambulance Service NHS Trust seen on 9 November in Wrexham. Number NA264 is seen wearing the dual Welsh/English lettering with 'Ambiwlans' written over the cab and 'Ambulance' on the bonnet.

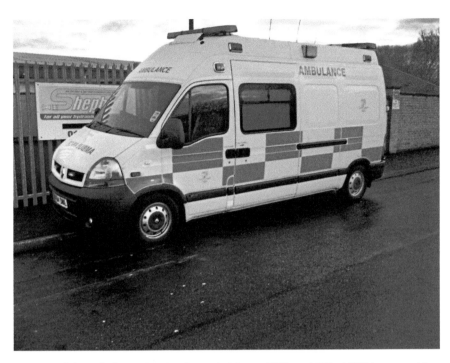

An ex-Welsh Ambulance Service Renault Master/Wilker, (OU54DWL), seen with a private operator on NHS support work on 8 December 2012. These ambulances still carried dual language interior signs.

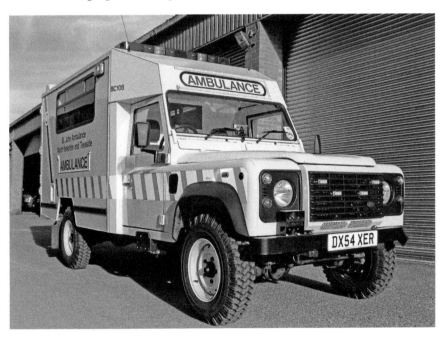

A 2004 Land Rover defender/M.M.B., (DX54XER) of St John Ambulance North Yorkshire and Teesside. When seen on 22 April 2008, this off-road ambulance was operational with the North Yorkshire and Teesside County as BC108.

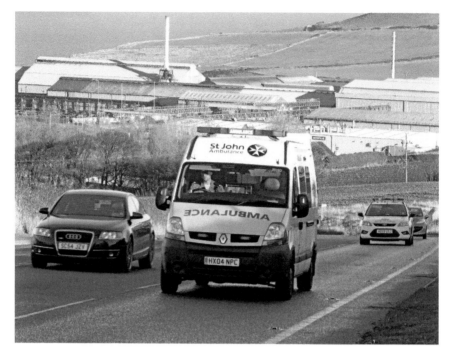

A St John Ambulance Renault Master/ATT Papworth, (HX04NPC), number JR110, working on NEAS support work, is followed by a NEAS Ford Focus/UVModular, (ND59USJ), climbing the A173 near Brotton on 10 November 2013.

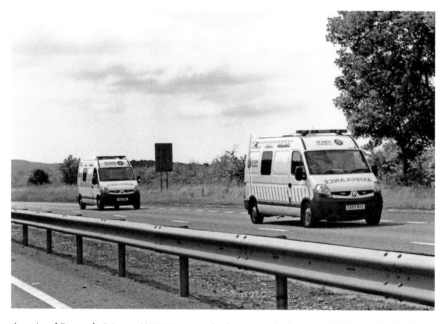

A pair of Renault Master/ATT Papworth-design ambulances of St John Ambulance northern area seen on the A19 near the Cleveland Tontine on 20 July 2016. (GX57BYG) from 2008, call sign JR134, leads 2010 (BX10BWK), VCS-built JR143, which is based at Thirsk.

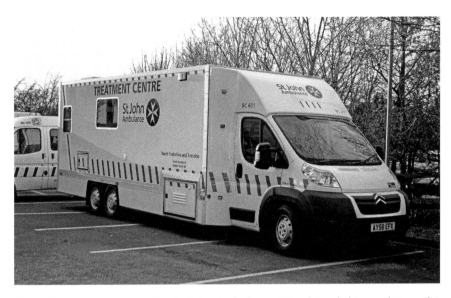

A mobile treatment centre for St John Ambulance (North Yorkshire and Teesside) seen on February 22 2009. This is a twin rear-wheeled vehicle on the Citroën Relay chassis, allocated call sign BC601, registration (AY58EFK). This was used at large events where there were no first-aid facilities available or additional treatment areas were needed.

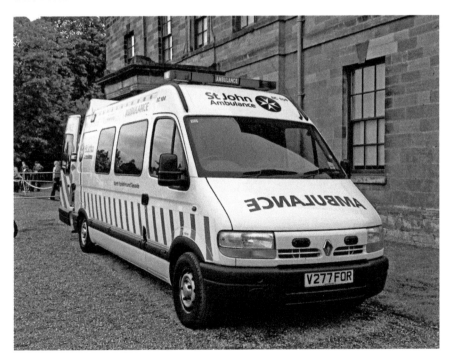

A Renault Master/ATT Papworth 'Crusader 900' of St John Ambulance North Yorkshire and Teesside, (V277FOR), call sign BC104. The design of these ambulances also allowed them to be used as mobile first-aid posts. This was seen being used as a first-aid post at Ormsby Hall at the 'Race for Life' event on 20 June 2009.

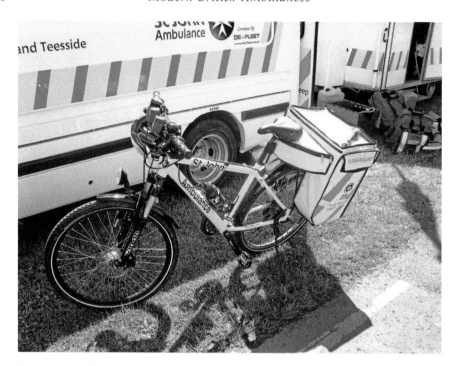

A mountain bike used as a cycle responder unit by St John Ambulance; one of a growing number when this was seen as it enabled a crowded event to have easier access to a patient, with equipment carried in the pannier bags on the back.

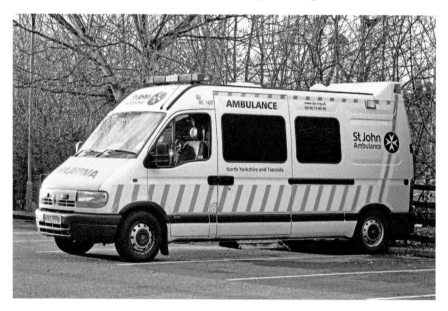

A 2002 Renault Master/VBB Papworth 'Crusader 900' ambulance, (HV02PFN) of St John Ambulance (North Yorkshire and Teesside), call sign BC107. This ambulance had been re-liveried with the new St John Ambulance logo. The new design has the St John Ambulance lettering and logo applied over the windscreen and the revision on the green and yellow chevron markings on the side.

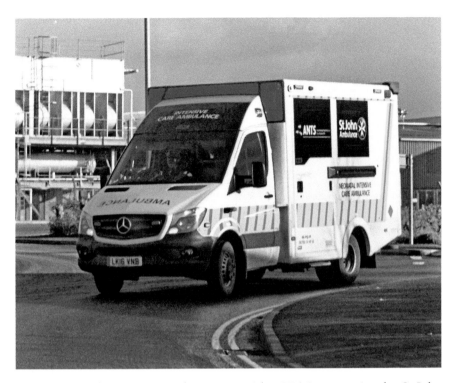

A 2016 Mercedes Benz 519 CdI Sprinter with a W.AS. conversion for St John Ambulance, number SR172, (LK16VNB), is seen at Kings Lynn, Norfolk, on 4 January 2017. This is a specialist Neonatal ambulance for carrying incubators for transfer between hospitals.

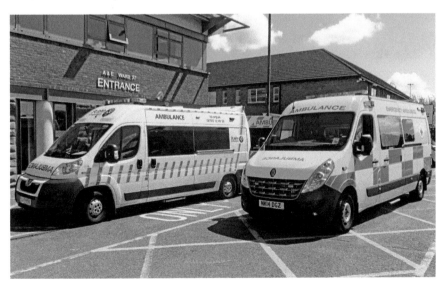

(LL13HSU), 2013 Peugeot Boxer/VCS conversion of St John Ambulance North East – call sign JR136 – stands next to (NL14DGZ), a 2014 Renault Master/W.A.S. of the British Red Cross Northern region. Both seen outside James Cook University Hospital A&E while on NEAS support.

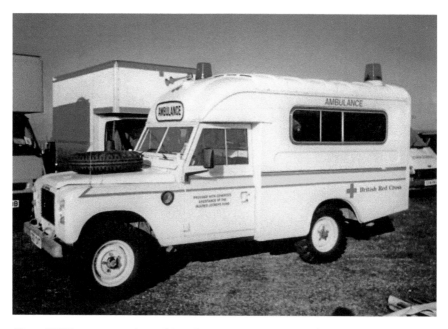

(D137DVT), a 1987 registered Land Rover Stage 1 V8/Herbert Lomas ambulance. Originally constructed for the Iranian Army, a trade embargo following the overthrow of the Shah left it sitting on Middlesbrough docks. In 1987 the British Red Cross purchased it for their Cleveland branch. In this photo (D137DVT) is seen at the 'Great North Run' on 6 October 2002. She was sold out of service in 2004. (Chris Playforth)

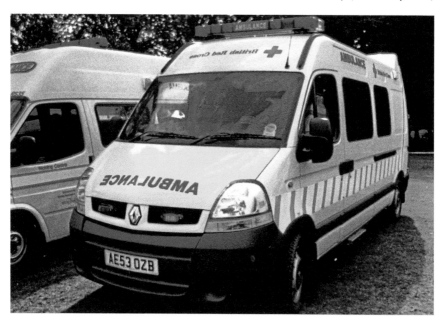

The British Red Cross used the Renault Master/ATT Papworth design, similar to the St John Ambulance design. These 'Challenger' models when first introduced used the yellow-and-red side-stripe colours in an alternating line pattern. This example from Surry branch, (AE53OZB), was seen when nearly new in August 2004.

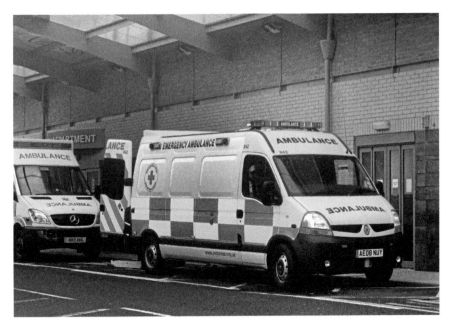

A 2008 Renault Master/M.M.B. of the British Red Cross County Durham, Teesside, Northumbria and Cumbria Branch fleet, (AE08NUY), number 842, is seen on NEAS support. Behind is North East Ambulance Service (NK11AHL), Mercedes Benz 519CdI/W.A.S., both seen outside the Emergency Department of the University Hospital of North Durham.

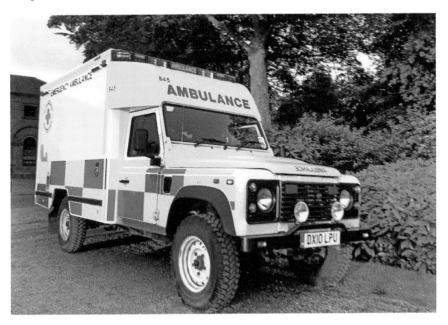

A 2010 Land Rover Defender/M.M.B. (Macclesfield Motor Bodies) of the British Red Cross Northern region, fleet number 845, (DX10LPU). This is seen at an event on 20 June 2014. For many years the British Red Cross used the Land Rover Defender/M.M.B. as the basis for its fleet of off-road-capable ambulances.

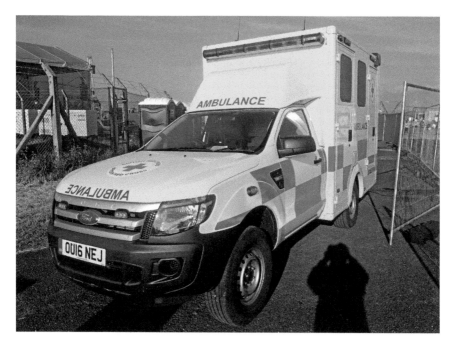

A 2016 Ford Ranger/W.A.S. ambulance conversion of the British Red Cross society Northern region, (OU16NEJ), seen while on a public duty on 28 May 2016 shortly after entering service. The Red Cross had previously used Land Rover Defender-based ambulances for their off-road fleet. (Chris Playforth)

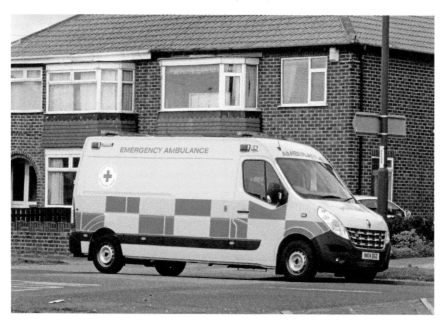

(NK14DGZ), 2014 Renault Master/W.A.S. of the British Red Cross seen on 17 April 2014 on NHS support work where it was attending a call. The Red Cross has been providing EMT level crews to NHS to respond to 999 and urgent calls under the control of the NHS services.

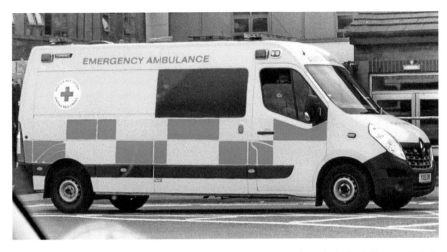

Another British Red Cross-operated Renault Master with a slightly different W.A.S. Conversion is this 2015 example, (YX15DYR), seen on NHS support work as a 999 response ambulance.

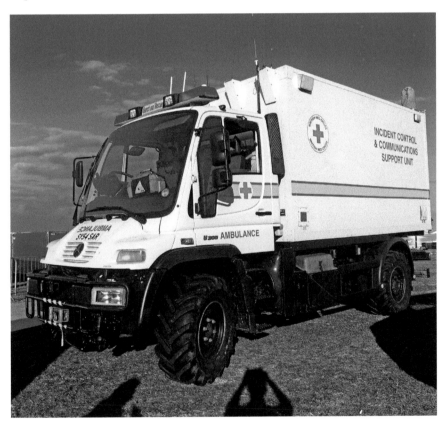

A 2014 Mercedes Benz Unimog U300 of the British Red Cross, (SY54SAR). This is operated in Scotland as a command and control communications support unit for use by the Red Cross and other emergency services. Seen here on 7 September 2014 at the 'Great North Run'. (Chris Playforth)

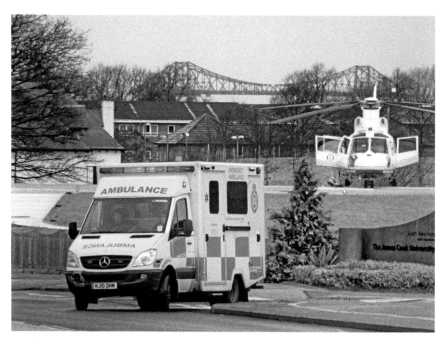

Land and air meet – A Mercedes Benz 519CdI Sprinter/WA.S. of North East Ambulance Service, (NJ10DHM), seen on the road. On the helipad behind, Aerospatiale AS365 Dauphin Helicopter, registration G-NHAA, the Great North Air Ambulance *Guardian of the North* can be seen.

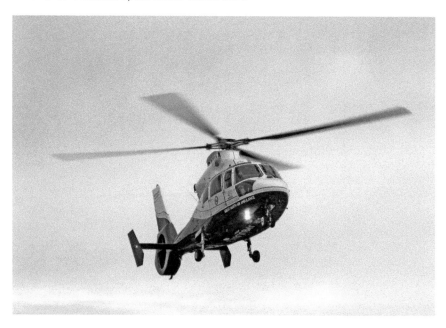

Aerospatiale AS365 Dauphin Helicopter, registration G-NHAA, the Great North Air Ambulance *Guardian of the North* is seen airborne in the sky above Middlesbrough on January 12 2014. This helicopter is based at Durham Tees Valley Airport near Darlington, County Durham.

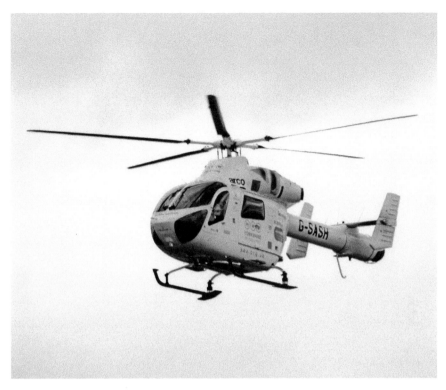

An MD 902 Explorer G-SASH of the Yorkshire Air Ambulance, *Helimed 99* flies over the Teesside sky on 18 July 2015. This is one of two helicopters operated by the Yorkshire Air Ambulance Service; the twin to this helicopter registration is G-CEMS.

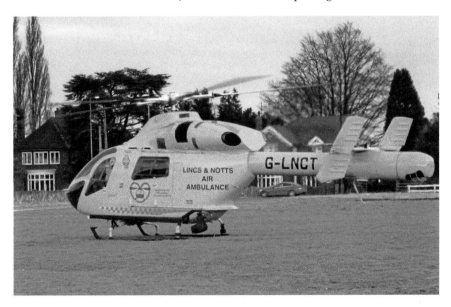

Seen outside Boston, Lincolnshire, G-LNCT – an MD902 Explorer Helicopter of Lincolnshire and Nottinghamshire Air Ambulance – prepares to take to the skies on February 15 2013. This is based at RAF Waddington near Lincoln.

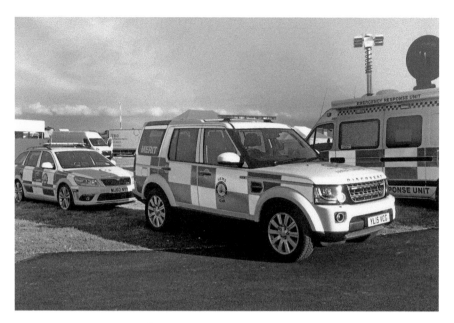

(YL15VCG), a 2015 Land Rover Discovery of the Great North Air Ambulance's Medical Emergency Response Incident Team (MERIT). (Chris Playforth)

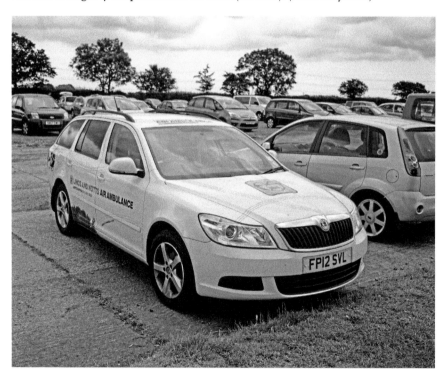

A Skoda Octavia of the Lincolnshire and Nottinghamshire Air Ambulance, (FP12SVL) is seen in Newark on 1 June 2015. This was used in a supporting role for the service. The helicopter Air Ambulance Services in England and Wales are charities that do not get funding from central government.

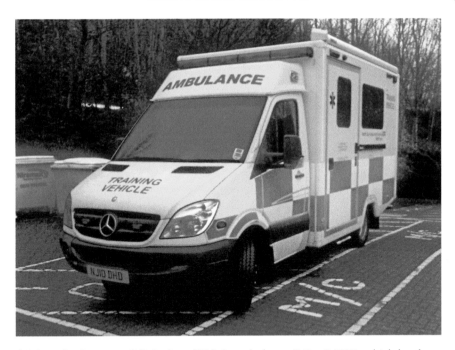

A Mercedes Benz 519CdI Sprinter/W.A.S. ambulance (NJ10DHD), which has been made specially to be a training ambulance for the North East Ambulance Service. This is seen at the Scottswood training centre, Newcastle-upon-Tyne, on 20 January 2012. It is used for practical training sessions.

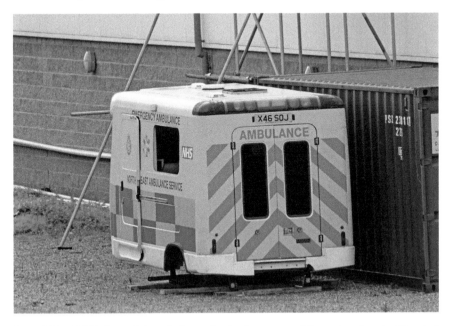

X46 SOJ a UVG 'Premia' ambulance body de-mounted from its chassis. Liveried as North East Ambulance Service, this was formerly a Renault Master of the West Midlands Ambulance Service. Seen sat in the grounds of Redcar College on 20 August 2015.

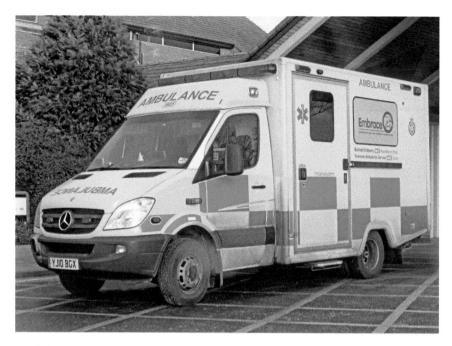

Yorkshire and Humber Infant and Children's Transport Service, EMBRACE, operated by the Sheffield Children's Hospital NHS Trust and Yorkshire Ambulance Service NHS Trust. The road service is operated on (YG10BGX), fleet number 1803, Mercedes Benz 519CdI Sprinter/W.A.S. ambulance, a specialist Paediatric ambulance.

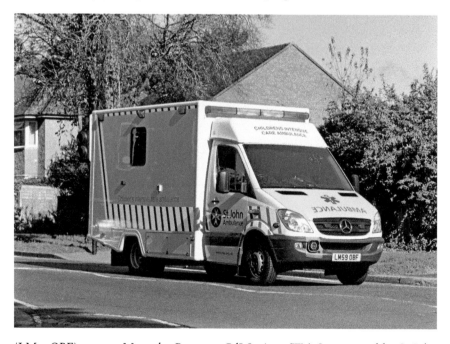

(LM59OBF), a 2009 Mercedes Benz 519CdI Sprinter/W.A.S., operated by St John Ambulance as a Children's Intensive Care ambulance. These are specially fitted out to carry incubators for hospital-to-hospital transfer.

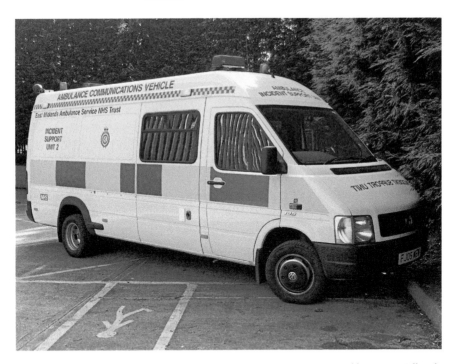

(FJ05WEW), a 2005 VWLT40/O&H communications unit operated by East Midlands Ambulance Service. This incident support unit of the Hazardous Area Response Team (HART) was seen at Alfreton in Derbyshire in 2012.

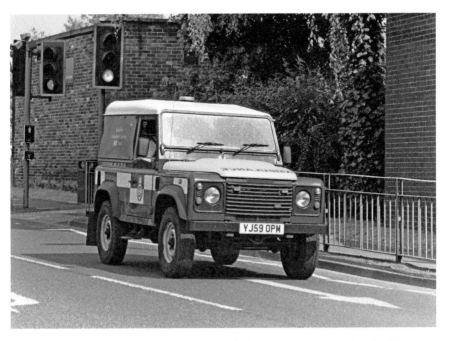

A Land Rover Defender of the Yorkshire Ambulance Service, (YJ59OPM). This is one of two operated by the Hazardous Area Response Team (HART) for use in North Yorkshire. It is seen in Northallerton, North Yorkshire.

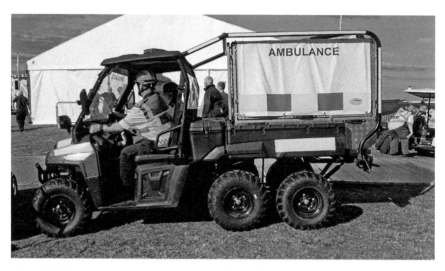

(SF59NZM), a 2010 Polaris Ranger 6x6 off-road specialist ambulance operated by the Hazardous Area Response Team (HART) of North East Ambulance Service. Seen at the 'Great North Run' on 11 September 2016. (Chris Playforth)

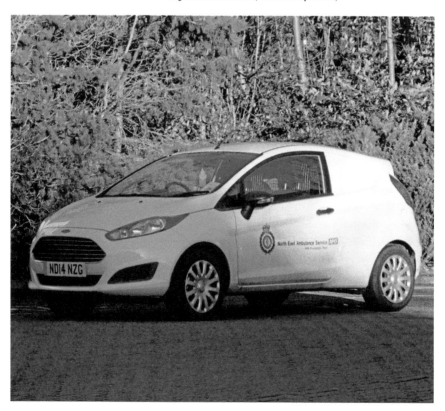

(ND14NZG), a 2014 Ford Fiesta, of the North East Ambulance Service training department. This is used for staff training in different stations and training centres as well as for commercial first-aid courses and transporting training materials. Seen on 15 January 2015 at the former Scottswood training centre, Newcastle-upon-Tyne.

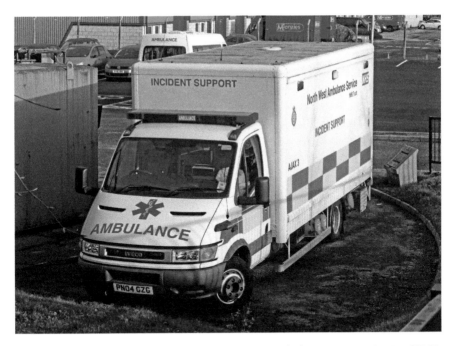

An Iveco Daily incident unit of the North West Ambulance Service, (PN04GZG). Designated fleet number AAJAX3, this is a Major Incident support unit and would be used in a mass casualty incident to transport additional equipment and shelters to the scene. Seen at Carlisle ambulance station, Cumbria.

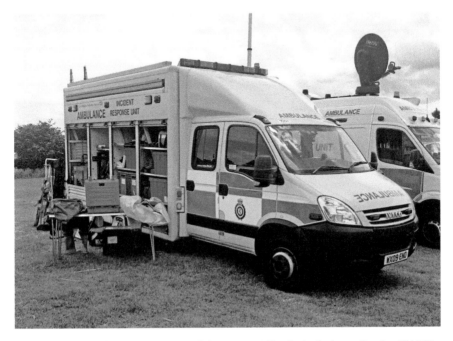

A 2009 Iveco Daily, (WX09ENO) of the East Midlands Ambulance Service HART – fleet number 1051. This Incident carrier is seen with some of the equipment that is carried inside it on display.

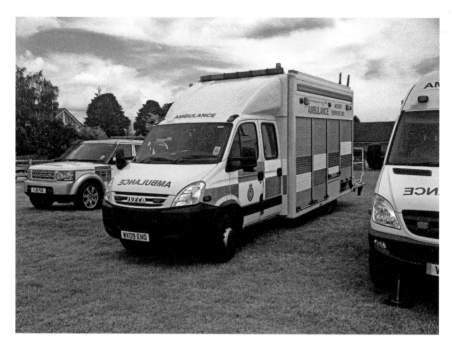

A 2009 Iveco Daily, (WX09ENO) of the East Midlands Ambulance Service HART – fleet number 1051. This photo shows the array of side lockers that have easy access to the equipment within. This class of carrier serve with all English ambulance services as part of the fleet of incident support units.

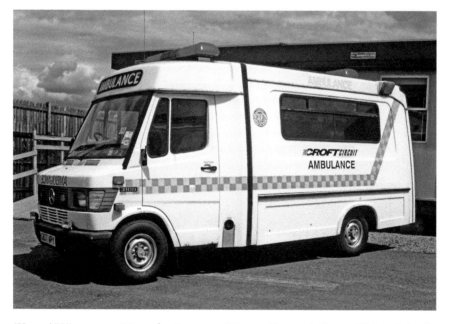

(K207APY), a 1993 Mercedes Benz 310/Customline ambulance. This originally started life with St John Ambulance Cleveland. It used to be number 107, attached to Middlesbrough (Central) division. This was photographed in 2009 when owned by Croft Race Circuit as one of their ambulances.

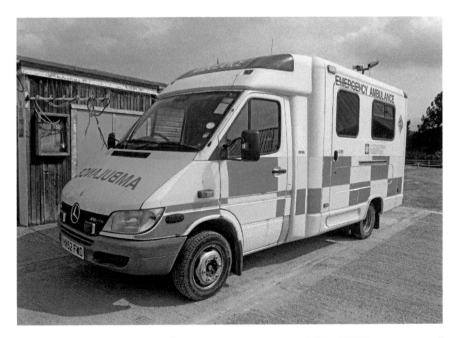

A 2002 Mercedes Benz 416CdI Sprinter/UVG 'Premia', (HN52FWO) was operated by MedicsUK in 2014 as the Boulby Potash mine-works ambulance. This ambulance was new to Hampshire Ambulance Service and also served with Conoco Phillips as a works ambulance to an oil refinery. It is stationed outside the mine medical facility to be used to take workers from the shaft to the medical room or helicopter landing pad if needed for transport off site in the event of an incident underground or around the surface plant.

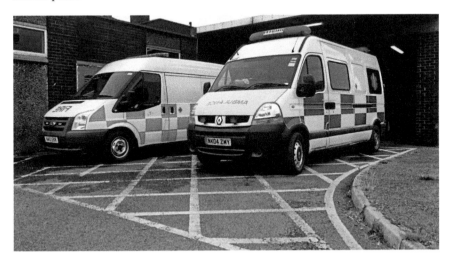

A double shot of the emergency services that serve the Lackenby steel plant site. These cover the former SSI blast furnace and steel production plants, the then Tata Steel-owned universal beam mill, and the AV Dawson-owned dispatch area. On the left is a 2010 Ford Transit, registration (NA10EKR), which is operated by the works' Fire and Rescue. Next to it is a 2004 Renault Master/Collet ambulance, registration (NK04ZMY).

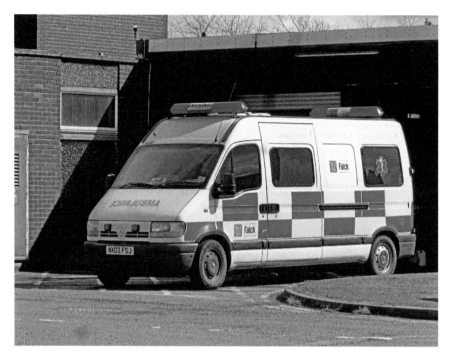

A 2003 Renault Master/Collet ambulance, (NX03FSJ) operated at the Lackenby steel works near Redcar. The Danish-based company Falck own this ambulance, which is seen at the site medical facility on 26 April 2016. (Stuart McKenzie)

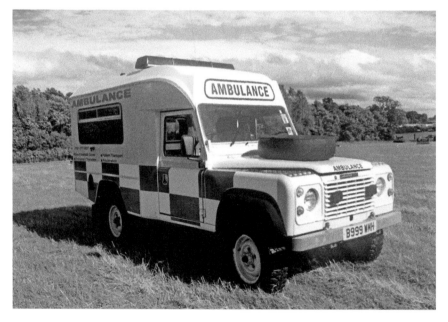

A 1985 Land Rover 110/Pilcher Greene ambulance, (B999WMH), running with a vanity plate. Originally registered in Birmingham, this was operated by Medical Services North East when seen on an equestrian event 18 August 2012 when the author was crewing the ambulance, which is now decommissioned.

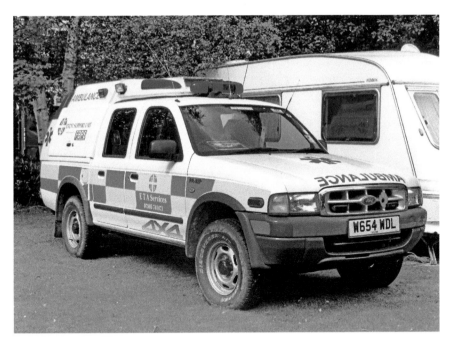

A 1999 Ford Ranger 4x4, (W654WTL). This was originally operated by West Midlands Ambulance Service as a response unit. It is seen on 24 August 2014 when being used as an event cover unit by ETA services. A similar design has been used by Fire and Rescue services.

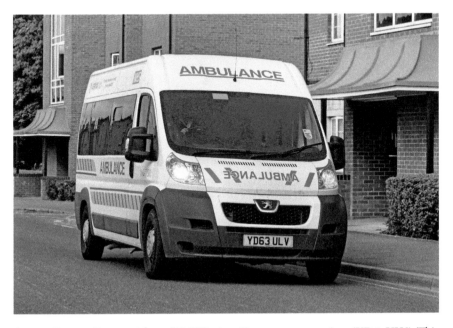

A 2013 Peugeot Boxer with an O&H Patient Transport conversion, (YD63ULV). This is operated by Arriva Ltd under a contract to provide all non-emergency out-patient ambulance transport. Arriva have these contracts in the North West, Midlands, and South West. This is seen leaving Gloucester hospital.

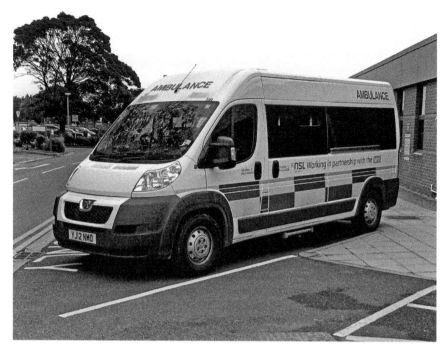

A 2012 Peugeot Boxer/O&H, (YJ12NMO). Operated by NSL care services, fleet number 2204 is seen on 5 October 2012 at Pilgrim Hospital Boston, Lincolnshire. This was a contract for providing non-emergency ambulance transport for the NHS.

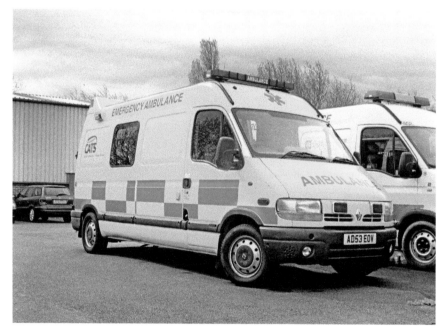

A 2003 Renault Master/ATT Papworth, (AD53EOV). A former Gloucestershire and later Great Western Ambulance Service ambulance, this is seen wearing the livery of Central Ambulance Training Services (CATS).

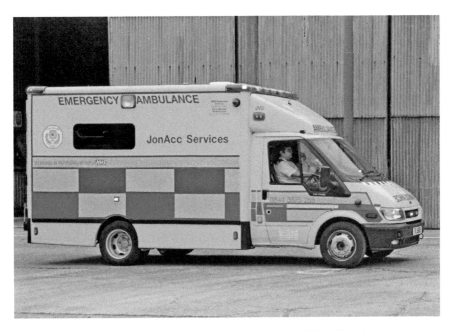

A 2006 Ford Transit/MacNeillie, (TIL 5963), fleet number JV3, of JonAcc services – an independent voluntary aid society based in Romford, Essex. They are seen operating an ex-Essex Ambulance Service ambulance wearing their distinctive livery. This has been used for events and their contract work to local hospitals and NHS ambulance support work.

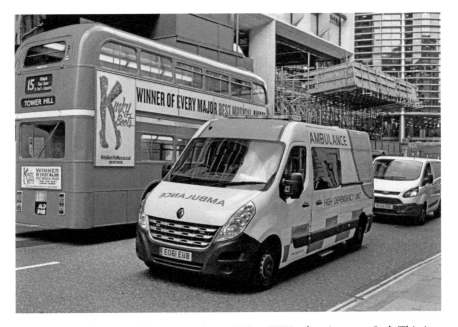

A 2011 Renault Master/PH conversions, (EO61 EUB) of caring4you Ltd. This is a high-dependency unit and is seen on Cannon Street, City of London, on 29 June 2016. This has a rather striking and colourful livery, differing from the often-seen 'Battenberg' green-and-yellow livery.

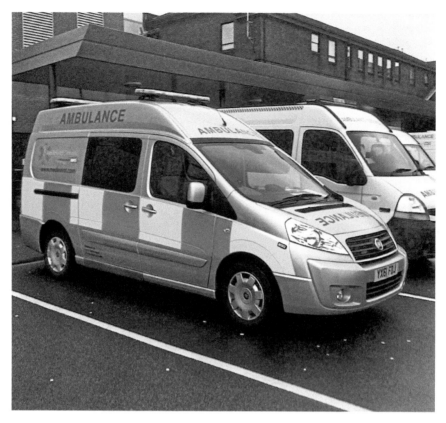

A Fiat conversion to an ambulance with Medivent Ltd seen at Kings Mill Hospital, Sutton-In-Ashfield, Mansfield, on 31 December 2012.

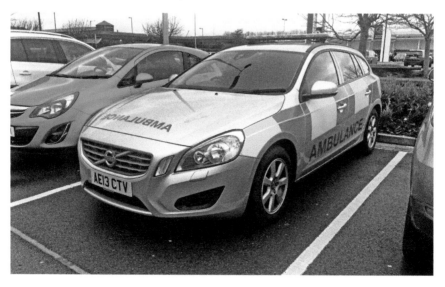

A 2013 Volvo V60 estate ambulance car, (AE13CTV), of Direct Medical Transport Limited of Carlton, Cleveland. Seen at Teesside Retail Park, Thornaby-on-Tees, on 4 January 2016.

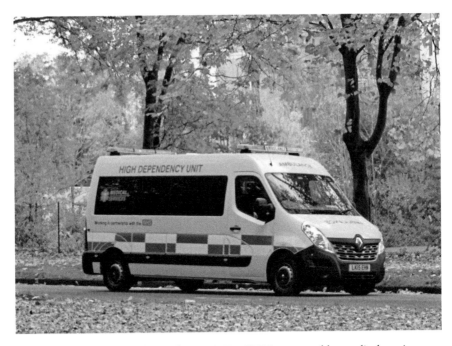

A 2015 Renault Master/Blue Light UK, (LK15EHN), operated by medical services as a high-dependency unit for NHS Urgent work. This has been given a customised livery to reflect the specialist work that this ambulance is used for and is seen while working in Birmingham.

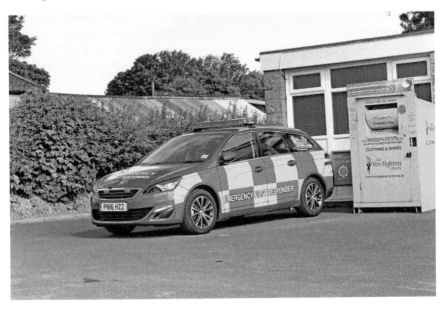

A joint venture between Yorkshire Fire and Rescue Service and Yorkshire Ambulance Service was of community co-responders where fire service crews would respond in rural areas as first responders to ambulance calls for serious cases. One example is this Peugeot 308 estate, (PN16HZZ), seen outside Lythe fire station, North Yorkshire, on 3 July 2016.

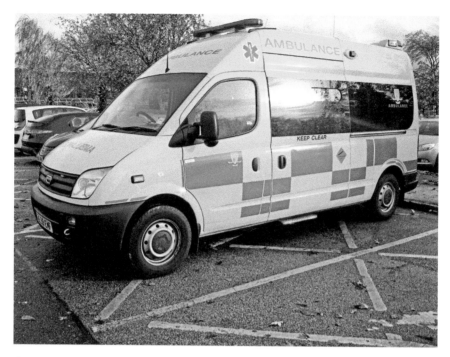

A 2010 LDV Maxus with Response SR conversion to an ambulance operated by Norvic ambulance and in use with Amvale 22 November 2012, while on a contract to the East Midlands Ambulance Service.

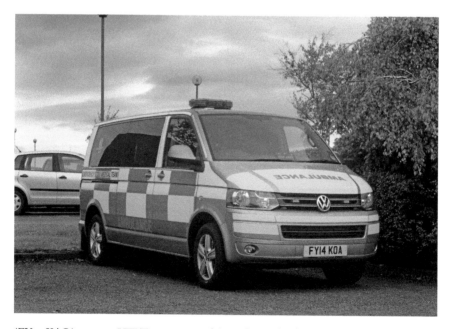

(FY14KAO), a 2014 VW Transporter of Amvale Medical Limited. These are used for the transporting of specialist organ transport teams and for the transport of organs to specialist transplant centres. A number of these are used for mental health transport as well. This is seen on 14 June 2014.

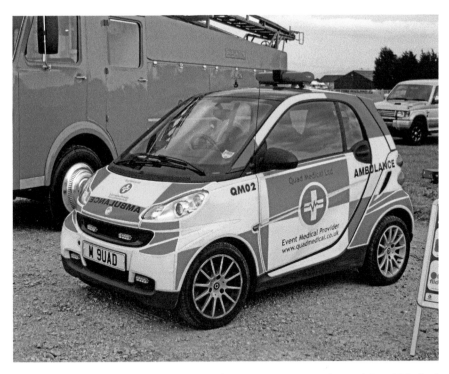

A rather unusual response ambulance is this Smart Car, (M9UAD), of Quad Medical Limited; an event medical provider seen at a display.

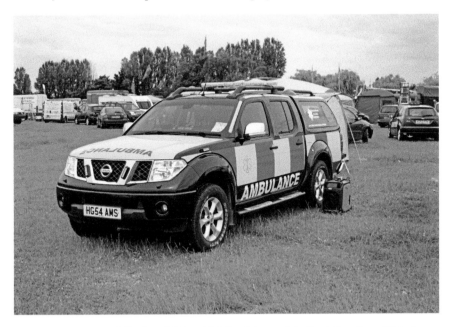

A 2008 Nissan Pathfinder, (HG54AMS) of Acute Medical Services. This has a personalised plate of the company name. These 4x4 response units are used by event companies for off-road response at events that van-derived ambulances would struggle to drive through.

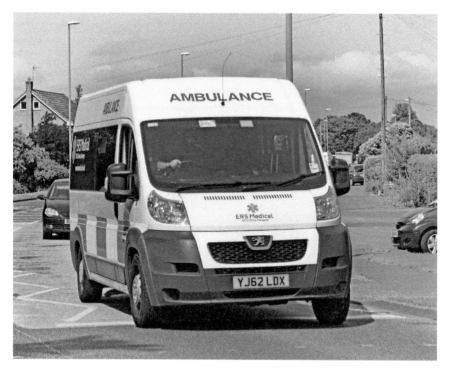

(YJ62LDX), a 2013 Peugeot Boxer/O&H Patient Transport ambulance of ERS Medical. This is seen Northallerton where it is used on a hospital discharge contract.

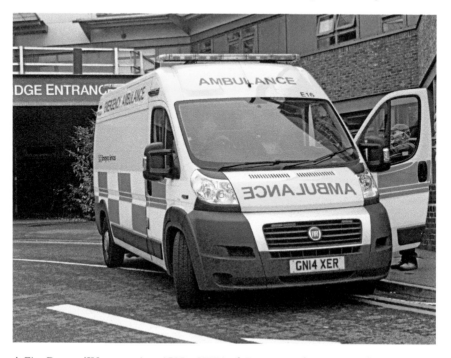

A Fiat Ducato/SV conversion, (GN14XER) of County Durham EMS. This is one of a number of ambulances used in contracts for the NHS